The Little Book of

MODERN GROOMING

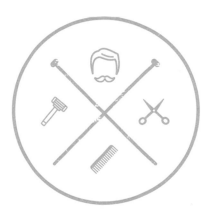

RUFUS CAVENDISH

circus

THE LITTLE BOOK OF MODERN GROOMING

This edition copyright © Summersdale Publishers Ltd, 2019
First published in 2018

Text by Chris Turton

Illustrations by Konstiantyn Federov

Cover images: Paper texture © Charcompix/Shutterstock.com; Razor and moustache man © M. Stasy/Shutterstock.com; Comb © Serhiy Smirnov/Shutterstock.com; Scissors © Viktoria Yams/Shutterstock.com; Divider © toonsteb/Shutterstock.com.

An Hachette UK Company
www.hachette.co.uk

Circus Books, an imprint of Summersdale Publishers Ltd
Part of Octopus Publishing Group Limited
Carmelite House
50 Victoria Embankment
LONDON
EC4Y 0DZ
UK

www.summersdale.com

Printed and bound in China

ISBN: 978-1-78783-297-8

Substantial discounts on bulk quantities of Summersdale books are available to corporations, professional associations and other organizations. For details contact general enquiries: telephone: +44 (0) 1243 771107 or email: enquiries@summersdale.com.

10 9 8 7 6 5 4 3 2 1

CONTENTS

INTRODUCTION – WHY BOTHER WITH GROOMING?

In essence, grooming is about giving time over to make yourself feel good – something that can be tricky in modern life. The bonus is that, as a result, you will look great. If you were the proud owner of a vintage sports car, chances are you'd want to clean, polish and maintain it, because it means a lot to you and you want to preserve it. As a result, it would run well and it would look awesome. Neglect it, and you won't be doing it justice. The message behind this book is that you deserve that sort of enthusiasm, care and attention – much more than a car or any other material object.

Grooming is by no means a recent invention. Men in ancient Egypt used black pigment to make their eyes look cat-like, Romans painted their heads to hide bald spots and in eighteenth-century France men wore powdered wigs and painted on beauty spots. The Victorians were famed for having tinctures and treatments for practically everything, not least facial hair, which included pomade, 'unguent' for the beard, and, of course, moustache wax.

This enthusiasm for grooming is arguably based solely around the desire to enhance one's outward appearance – the Victorian gentleman might have thought it unseemly to appear in public with unkempt facial hair, but would have been ignorant of the fact that if he could acquire some coconut oil and apply it to his face, its antioxidant properties would be great for his skin. And that's where today's man is at an advantage. Scientific research has revealed countless new ways of looking after ourselves and has shown us not only the cosmetic but also the physical and mental benefits of doing so. Basic hygiene is a given – floss and you avoid tooth problems, trim your nails and you avoid ingrowing nails, wash your hair regularly with anti-dandruff shampoo and you avoid a flaky scalp. Grooming, of the kind illustrated in this book, takes this principle to a level where you can get downright fancy with ways to enhance how you look and feel, at the same time developing a positive, self-caring attitude. And the more you invest in grooming, the more you'll get out of it.

- Hair -

Your hair is arguably the most groom-worthy feature of your body, so that's where we'll start. The great thing about hair is that it can be trimmed, teased and tied pretty much at will – you can make it a style statement or treat it as something to be kept in check. (Your approach will probably vary depending on the area of the body in question.) But just because it's a really obvious area to focus on doesn't mean to say it's that straightforward!

- The Head -

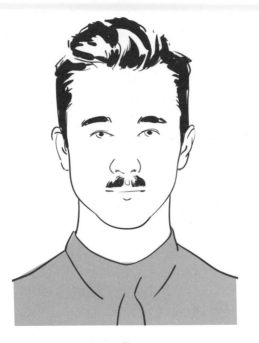

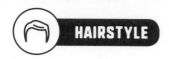

Haircuts begin as something your parents force upon you, like going to the dentist or eating your vegetables, but by the time you're your own man, you adopt your own style. Choosing a hairstyle might sound simple – you'll try many throughout your lifetime, some inspired by trends, some by practicality – but have you ever taken the time to think about what hairstyle you *should* have? You might love the idea of a classic quiff, frohawk or undercut, but you should consider two things before you jump in: (1) is the style you're going for practically achievable? and (2) will that style suit your face?

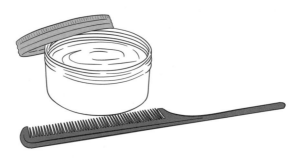

HAIR TYPES

Assessing your hair type is the first step to style success. The list below is a rough guide to what hair type is generally compatible with what style:

✂ Straight – often needs a lot of work to create texture and volume, so go for a no-nonsense classic short cut such as a simple side parting. Or try a choppy top with texture cut in, with short sides. On similar lines, you could go for an undercut with a clean, swept-back style on top. When worn too long, this hair type is likely to look limp and unattractive.

PROPER PARTING

If you're going for a part in your hair, take the time to find where it naturally occurs. Parting it on the natural side will ensure your hair sits properly once styled (although, as always, a ton of product and effort can defy gravity). An easy way is to brush your hair forward, onto your forehead, and look in a mirror to see where a part is occurring. You can also use a couple of mirrors to observe your crown – if the hair is circling in a clockwise direction, part your hair on the left side of your head.

✂ Wavy – waves are enviable, as you will have natural texture and volume, but can also make it a challenge to control and shape your hair. Let the waves do their thing and grow your hair long enough for them to show; long hair will look great, as will mid-length hair with short back and sides (but be sure it's thinned out on top, to avoid the mop look). Accept that your look is a little untamed and let go of the idea of tight, tidy styles (unless you want to spend your life using straighteners).

✂ Curly – like wavy hair, curls have natural style. This hair type is often thicker and has a lot of structure, which can be a bonus in terms of achieving volume and shape, but also means it can be hard to style. As with wavy hair, some length for looser curls is preferable. For tighter, dense curls, hairstyling becomes more akin to sculpture; this hair type has texture even at very short length, so a buzz cut will suit just as well as a high fade with some length on top. You could experiment with twists and dreads, curls or a flat top.

✂ Thinning – if you're completely lacking on top, you can experiment with facial hair to make the most of the hair elsewhere on your head. Check out the section on The Face on p.39. If you're working with thinning hair, there are various options, depending on where your hair is lacking. A buzz cut is a smart option if you have fairly even coverage, and it's a standard for balding men, since it reduces everything to the same length. For receding hairlines, you could try an Ed Sheeran brushed-forward-but-messy style, but this amounts to a kind of combover, which can look awkward if the wind blows in the wrong direction!

Admittedly, there are ways to defy your hair type. There are products and techniques that you can use to help you achieve the look you're after, in spite of your natural type – but grooming isn't always about spending hours on your style; it's about making what you've got better, and being savvy about the time you spend.

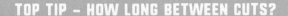

TOP TIP – HOW LONG BETWEEN CUTS?

There is no set rule about how often you should visit the hairdresser – it depends entirely on your circumstances and your style. A reasonable average is every four weeks, but this can be stretched if you have a longer cut that is less reliant on intensive styling.

FACE SHAPE

When it comes to face shape, in most cases you'll want to balance out your natural face type with something that contradicts it. This list will give you an idea of what to consider:

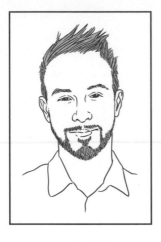

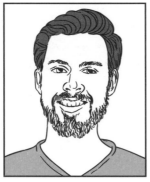

◀ OVAL FACE

Not too wide, not too long. As such, you want a style that doesn't go one way more than it does the other; not too high or too wide – you want to retain that oval shape. Shorter styles are best – short back and sides, with a little more length on top. Buzz cuts and fringes will make your face look rounder, which isn't recommended, but long hair should still work.

SQUARE FACE ▶

Adding height to a more evenly proportioned face is one way to ensure you look good. As opposed to a round face, a square face has natural angles, so you can actually balance the square with a softer-edged, rounder hairstyle – so closely cropped hair works well too. Styles that creep onto the forehead – fringes or short dreads – will also look good. You can pretty much do what you want!

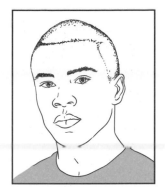

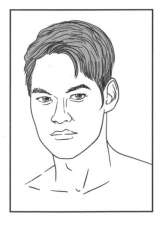

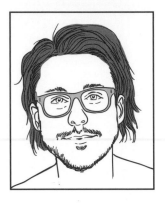

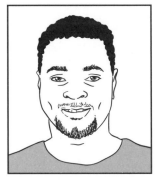

◀ ROUND FACE

Making an oval out of the round shape is the aim here, so you'll want to subtract width and add height. Go for a short cut on the sides and some length on top (but short enough to style your hair 'up' in a quiff or messy peaks or twists). Again, avoid buzz cuts and fringes. Long hair is doable but it needs to have some uneven structure to it, to break up the round face shape, so a parting might help. You can also lengthen the round shape at the other end and grow a beard.

DIAMOND FACE ▶

This face type takes the basic shape of an upside-down triangle in its lower half, so the chin will make the shape come to a point at the bottom. For this face shape, balance out the point at the bottom with a point at the top, so a messy, peaked style – maybe even a mohawk – will work well. So will a slick-back style or a textured crop with some of the hair forming a bit of a fringe to soften the pointed lines of the face.

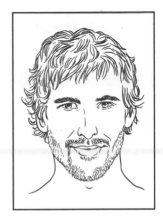

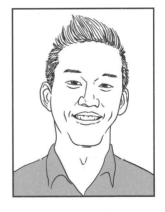

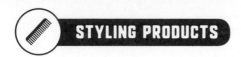

STYLING PRODUCTS

Once you've found your cut, you need to put the work in to keep the style. A key thing to consider is how much time you want to spend on your hair each day. Do you have time to blow-dry, brush, style and finish your hairdo every day, or are you looking for a good-quality product that will sort your hair out with a quick application and some freeform hand-styling? Of course, you can do both, but it's worth thinking it over before you plunge into the vast universe that is men's hairstyling.

CHOOSING THE RIGHT STYLING PRODUCT FOR YOU

As with your haircut, enhancing your style will involve two main considerations: (1) will the product work with the natural condition of your hair? and (2) will the product allow you to achieve what you're after? Ultimately, both points will require a bit of trial and error, but a rule of thumb is that you don't want anything with a thickening effect if you have thick hair; and you don't want anything with a thinning effect if you have fine hair. At the same time, if your hair has excess natural oil in it, you don't want to add more; if your hair is dry, introducing a moisturizing product will make it more manageable. The trick is to balance out what you have – and if in doubt, just ask your hairdresser.

TOP TIP – BEFORE YOU REACH FOR THE PRODUCT

If you know your style will need to be blow-dried into shape – if it requires serious height, for instance – skip ahead to p.27 for some advice on how to work some magic with the dryer first.

✎ Wax – this is the ideal, all-round product. A lot of products, even those that aren't called 'wax', will contain an element of wax. It generally gives a medium to high hold, can have a matte or shiny finish, and is excellent for creating volume and texture, retaining flexibility for reshaping. It's not intended for uniform, every-hair-in-place styles, and it's best shaped with fingers rather than a brush or comb. It doesn't get on too well with thick and/or curly hair, since it's quite thick itself, but more so with straight or wavy hair, especially if it's fine.

Pomade – this old-fashioned favorite has had a renaissance thanks to a rise in the popularity of 'classic' styles like the pompadour. Pomade, like cream, is somewhat nourishing, so is suitable for thicker hair. It will also spread easily through coarse hair and tight curls. They give the best hold and definition for longer, finer hair, though, and provide the perfect finish for a sleek, slicked-back look, without any actual greasiness. Products like this go hand in hand with a comb and are ideal for sweeping, even styles, where every hair is neatly in place.

The key to applying product is this – start small and build it up if necessary. Yes, there is something to be said for the 'pea-sized amount' recommended on most packaging. Rub the product in your hands vigorously and brush the surface of your hair all over before running your fingers through from root to tip. If you've put too much on, use a towel and rough your hair up to remove it before you think about giving up and washing it out.

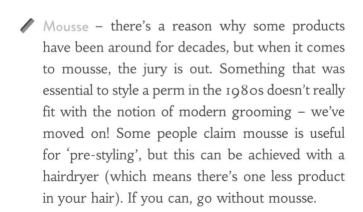

Mousse – there's a reason why some products have been around for decades, but when it comes to mousse, the jury is out. Something that was essential to style a perm in the 1980s doesn't really fit with the notion of modern grooming – we've moved on! Some people claim mousse is useful for 'pre-styling', but this can be achieved with a hairdryer (which means there's one less product in your hair). If you can, go without mousse.

🖌 Gel – this might not be the same as products from days gone by, which gave you hair that could double up as a high-impact safety helmet, but the consistency of gel, and how it sets your style, just seems counterintuitive if you want a less 'processed' look – and it reduces fingers-through-the-hair-ability. Used sparingly, it can be a useful quick-fix remedy, but it's not as versatile as a wax or clay.

🖌 Relaxers – if you're working with tight curls and coils, you might want to use something to relax and soften the naturally tight condition of your hair to achieve a more workable and flowing look.

🖌 Cream – as this has a lighter consistency than wax, it will be suitable for thicker hair, as well as finer hair, when used moderately. It will have a medium to low hold, so it's better if you're after a less formal look, and perhaps have longer hair that you just want to keep in check and de-frizz. It often contains hair-enriching elements, so it's great for dry hair as well as tight curls and coils.

🖋 Putty and Fibre – these two will usually give high hold and low (or no) shine. As opposed to wax, they might be more workable on application. Putty is good for shorter styles. Fibre is one of the best options for guys with thicker hair, as it can help wrangle your style into place without too much effort. It's not suitable for combing, though.

🖋 Paste and Clay – both of these products often give a medium hold and low shine. They tend to be fairly thick in consistency, but not so much that they will detract from thicker hair. They are good all-round, middle-of-the-road options. If your hair is thinning, these products are great, since a matte finish will absorb light, which has the effect of making your hair look thicker.

🖋 Finishing products – you might be aiming for a style that requires a lot of work – maybe some blow-dry styling, followed by a dab of base product like pomade to smooth out your hair and give it a healthy shine. But if you don't fix your hair into place, especially if you have finer hair, your style could fall flat.

This is where finishing products come in. The most common one for the scenario above would be hairspray – just a little for that extra hold. There are products to boost volume, add gloss and de-frizz, but these tend to be more appropriate for long hair (6 inches or more). It seems the longer your hair is, the more attention and nurturing it needs; so if this is you, take some time to find a product that suits (but maybe start with a shampoo that does some of the work for you – see p.30).

TOP TIP – HAIR-EMERGENCY HACK

On days when there's moisture in the air, your hair can get messed up pretty quickly. If this happens, and you don't have any of your usual products to hand, search out the hand cream. You might have

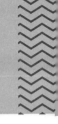

some in the restrooms at work, you might be able to borrow some from a friend or colleague – that part's up to you. Use it like you would any styling product to shape and tame your hair. It's a quick fix, but will save you from looking scruffy!

 BRUSHES AND COMBS

If you're looking for a more structured, uniform style, a brush or comb is indispensable. Brushes are good for getting the basic style in place and adding volume (often while blow-drying), and combs can help with the finishing touches after you've applied your styling product.

Here's a summary of what to go for, depending on your hair type:

HAIR TYPE	RECOMMENDED BRUSH STYLE
Curly (loose)	A wide-toothed comb will help give order to your locks
Curly (tight)	In general, a wide-toothed comb with rounded teeth will style and help reduce damage; an afro comb/pick is a classic option for a more dense style
Fine	A soft-bristle brush will help give volume and avoid damage
Thick	A brush with stiff bristles is the way to go
Medium	This hair type is arguably the least troublesome, but you will still do well to use a stiff-bristled brush for general styling

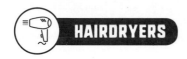

HAIRDRYERS

If you naturally lean towards a more no-nonsense hair-styling routine, you might be happy to give hairdryers a miss altogether. However, if you have long locks, or your hair is less inclined to behave and settle into a style (especially a voluminous one), you should consider it. High-end hairdryers will promise damage-reduction technology, which might be worth shelling out for if you're going to make blow-drying a daily thing. But whether your dryer is bargain-basement or top-of-the-line, you need to know how to use it.

1. Remove as much moisture as possible from your hair with a towel, using a scrunching action.

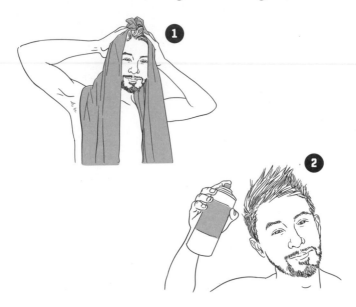

2. Add heat-protection spray for extra protection before drying.

3. Start drying on a low setting, slowly building up the temperature (flash-drying your hair is sure to damage it).

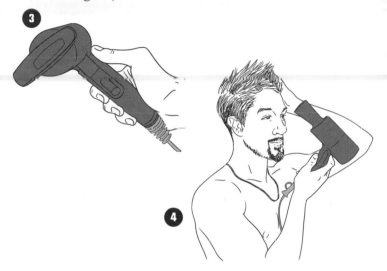

4. With shorter hair, you could use your fingers or a brush to start persuading your style into place (in between drying, not at the same time!). Nailing the brushing-while-blowing technique might be too fussy, so this technique is a good compromise.

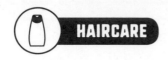 **HAIRCARE**

The first step in your style routine actually begins in the shower. Using a shampoo that complements your hair type will give your hairdo the best possible start. There is some research to suggest that daily washing is detrimental to the condition of your scalp and hair, but if you're determined to get your grooming groove on, and use hair products on a regular basis, it's hard to see how you can avoid it.

For fine hair, something that adds volume and nourishment (amino acids and keratin) will be beneficial. Thick (and dry) hair, on the other hand, needs no help with volume; in fact, it probably needs relaxing, so moisturizing shampoos will help. The same goes for tightly curled hair – natural oil (sebum) has a hard time dispersing from scalp to hair tip, so moisturizing shampoos are a big plus. Oily hair is not necessarily something you can fix with washing. It's a result of excess oil production, which is something your body controls. In this instance, washing your hair every other day can help rebalance the condition of your hair and scalp. For when you do shampoo, there are 'rebalancing' formulas out there for you to try.

GO *NATUREL* – HAIR MOISTURIZER

There are all sorts of moisturizing serums on the market, promising to nourish your hair to perfection, but this is one area where you can save a little money. Ditch the processed products that offer natural ingredients and go straight to the source. Combine four parts shea butter (softened in a microwave) with three parts aloe vera gel to create a fresh, luxuriant hair mask. Apply liberally after washing and drying your hair. Store in a cool, dry place.

A HEALTHY SCALP

It's easy to forget about your scalp when considering haircare – after all, it's kind of hiding most of the time! But the scalp can be the root cause (see what I did there?) of various hair issues. We've already mentioned oily hair, where the scalp is producing excess sebum, but there are a number of other common problems that are worth addressing. Excess oil, ironically, can lead to dandruff, which is a long-term condition, but can be controlled with medicated shampoos.

You might also experience a flaky scalp as a result of a reaction to a product you've used. If you notice itching or flakes where none have been previously, take some time to consider if it's something you've introduced yourself. Common irritants can include sodium lauryl/laureth sulphate, cocamide DEA, TEA or MEA, and cocamidopropyl betaine.

SATURATE AND STIMULATE

Aside from avoiding irritants, there are a few essential things you can do to care for your scalp:

X Wash hair with tepid water, which reduces the drying-out effect.

X Nourish your scalp with a conditioner.

X Stimulate your follicles with a scalp massage (you can do this yourself!).

X Protect your hair against sun damage (find a hat that suits you for the hottest days).

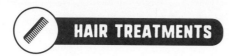

HAIR TREATMENTS

You might be in a situation where no matter what style you wear or what product you use, you're unhappy about your hair. You might want to change the color (out of preference, or in an attempt to hold back the grey) or you might simply want more of it. Here are a few pointers.

DYEING YOUR HAIR

If you're set on changing your natural hair color, there are a few things to keep in mind. Consider if the new color suits your skin tone. Your skin and natural hair color share the same base pigments, so if you stray too far your new color will clash. If you have black or brown hair, you will have 'warm' undertones in your skin (orange, brown, gold or orange-based red) and so your new color should have an element of gold or honey color. If you have blond hair, you will have 'cool' undertones like blue, green, pink or blue-based red, so your new color should have an element of black, white-blonde or auburn.

Don't forget, though, if you have prominent eyebrows you'll have to treat them too!

MANAGING GREY HAIR

Some men are shocked to the core by a single grey hair and others learn to love them. Greying is a natural process, so it's nothing to be embarrassed about. You only need to look at celebs like George Clooney or George Lamb to realize that being a silver fox can be a winning option. However, if you're determined to ease the transition, here are some tips to get you going:

✂ Tweeze as you please – there's no harm in removing the odd grey, if that's all it is.

✂ Cover and conceal – a root concealer can take care of smaller grey patches.

✂ Trim and proper – grey hair is thicker than non-grey, so opt for a shorter hairstyle.

✂ Shampoo and shine – switch to a grey-hair shampoo to remove yellow tones, which can look unappealing, and keep your grey hair looking vibrant.

THINNING ON TOP

If you're thinning on top, you might feel like you're losing your mojo – after all, hair is associated with virility (even if there is little, scientifically, to back this up). On the other hand, you might choose to accept it, and work with it.

If you're determined to fight the fading hairline and if male pattern baldness is the cause, be aware that there is no current cure, so the best you can do is slow it down. The most famous over-the-counter solution is minoxidil (e.g. Rogaine), which is said to stimulate growth when applied to the scalp. Then there is the extreme end of the scale – hair transplants. To many people this will be a step too far (after all, there are many Hollywood A-listers who have been ridiculed for their efforts), and of course it's heinously expensive.

Working with what you have (and we're not talking combovers!) might be the best place to start. Get a haircut that complements your hair – if it's thin all over, consider a buzz cut; if you've got some length and decent coverage, rough layers can add depth and texture. Facial hair is a way to focus your style on places your hair is still thriving.

You can also make various simple lifestyle changes that might help – more of which in the well-being section (p.136).

GO *NATUREL* - HAIR LOSS REMEDIES

One method is to extract the juice from an onion (grate it and then put the pulp into muslin or a clean handkerchief and squeeze out the juice), rubbing it into the scalp twice a day for 30 minutes, then washing out. A less pungent idea is to apply aloe vera gel which is said to promote healthy growth. These remedies can be hit or miss, but worth a try for such a low cost.

- The Face -

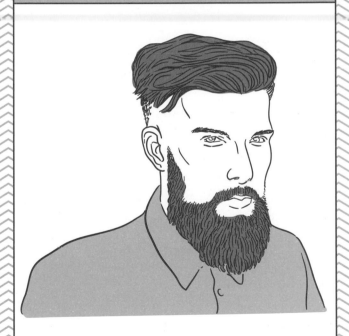

For some guys, facial hair is little more than something to be carefully removed as part of a daily routine, while others relish the thought of breaking out the wax and comb to tend to their elaborate moustache or flocculent beard. The latter offers more opportunities for grooming, but it's also yet another thing to look after, so we'll start this chapter by looking at the most basic option: shaving.

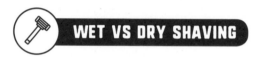

WET VS DRY SHAVING

Unbelievably, cropping facial hair with a sharp edge dates back to prehistoric times, so it might well be the first grooming practice ever! Early man might have smelled like a woolly mammoth's rear end, but you better believe his facial-hair game was on point. But, to get back to the subject at hand, a razor, being the most common way to wet-shave, is still as popular as it has ever been. Straight 'cut-throat' razors, as used in the 1800s, are sometimes still called upon today, but most men opt for the modern version of the 'safety razor', which has now evolved into the disposable 'cartridge' razor.

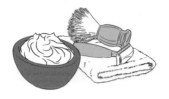

◄ WET SHAVING

This results in a super-smooth finish, because of the closeness of the shave and also because it's exfoliating, so it removes dead skin cells as well as hair. The biggest con is probably the cost of new cartridges (or new razors, if you use disposables), and their constant 'reinvention' by the addition of yet another blade justifying a higher price. A slightly less convenient, but ultimately cheaper option is to shell out for an old-fashioned-style safety razor and master the art of one-blade shaving. The blades for these are double-edged and infinitely cheaper and can be recycled (though you will need to dispose of them as sharps/biohazard) – and you'll gain extra man-points. With both options you run the risk of cuts (though that's pretty hard to do with a multi-blade cartridge) and skin irritation (razor burn – see p.87, in Skin, for more info).

DRY SHAVING ▶

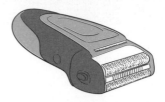

An electric shaver is your other option. Since the original US patent, submitted by John F. O'Rouke in 1898, electric shavers have gone all hi-tech. An electric shaver has a high cost at the outset, but if maintained it will give years of mess-free shaving. Except, you can't replicate that spotless, wet-shave feel, and some might find that certain shavers don't catch many hairs (though this is usually because you're using a bad shaver or you're doing something slightly wrong). There's also the maintenance factor – not so hard if you have an expensive self-cleaning bit of kit – and the charging. Charging shouldn't be a challenge, but somehow forgetting to do it is very easy.

Of course, the choice is yours, but if a well-conditioned, hair-free face is what you're after, you can't do much better than a wet shave.

EYEBROWS, NOSE AND EARS

Once you've taken care of the unwelcome hairs on your face, you will want to turn your attention to the less obvious, often neglected areas. We're talking eyebrows, nose and ears. All three of these areas mostly need the hair trimmed or removed, as opposed to conditioned, but you need to aim to make this a habit.

EYEBROWS

Unibrows, like unicorns, are something of a rare sight among grown men – tweezing out the hairs that grow between the two brows is often the very least a guy will do to keep them in check. But there's more to brows than what meets in the middle. To keep them looking sharp, follow these basic steps:

✂ Brush your brows with a cheap, clean toothbrush or a moustache comb, if you have one.

✂ Trim any extra-long or out-of-place hairs with some small scissors (nail scissors will do).

✂ Brush and repeat.

✂ Get your pluck on for hairs that are growing outside of the main brow area – pull them out in the direction they grow.

NOSE

If your face is perfectly preened, but your nasal passages look like two hairy caterpillars have made them their home, your good work has been wasted. That said, your nasal hair does have a legitimate function – it's a barrier against microbes – so you don't want to lose it completely. Keeping it in check is the thing to do. Like most grooming operations, you can go manual or automatic. Using a multi-purpose pair of small scissors, good for all types of fine-hair adjustments, is the budget option; if you're keen to splash out, buy a multi-function trimmer, not just a nose-hair trimmer. Trim protruding hairs and thin out the passages – just don't annihilate the whole lot. Plucking will bring tears to your eyes, and potentially do some damage, so it's not advisable.

EARS

Rogue hairs can sprout up from around the ear canal as well as on the surface of the outer ear. They might be light and downy, in which case perhaps you can live with them, but if they start to develop some thickness you will want to remove them. And removal is the game, so tweezing and waxing (by a professional) are two sensible, if slightly painful options. If your trimmer has a suitable attachment, you could buzz away the offending hairs, but this won't last as long as when you tweeze or wax. Certain barbers (often Turkish, but the trend is picking up) will offer a flame-based removal method, whereby the hairs are singed away – painless and theatrical!

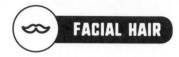 **FACIAL HAIR**

Grooming today has become synonymous with moustaches, beards and 'designer' stubble, which some people might simply not like the idea of. To grow and maintain facial hair is an effort and perhaps there's no room for that in your routine (or in your budget). But for others, facial hair is another way to express their style.

WILL IT SUIT ME?

Like your hairstyle, there are some styles of facial hair that simply won't suit you as well as others (or at all), so it's worth considering this before you stop shaving. As with your haircut, face shape has a role to play, and the idea is pretty much the same – balance out what you've got. Here's a summary of what might work:

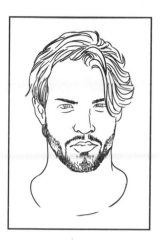

◄ OVAL

most styles will work,
but try a horseshoe
moustache or
short, full beard.

ROUND ►

add some angles and
length with a goatee
or longer full beard
with short sides.

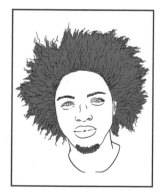

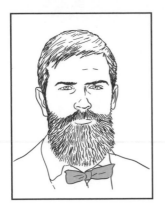

◄ SQUARE

emphasize your manly
jaw with a tidy, short
moustache or soften
it with a rounder-
shaped beard.

DIAMOND ►

soften the point and fill
in the angular bottom
portion of your face
with a full, long beard
or heavy stubble.

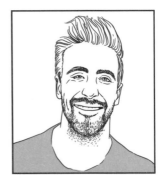

Note: this is obviously just a rough guide. You're at
liberty to grow anything you like, and the best way to
know if it suits you is to try it. If it looks silly, simply
shave it off!

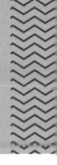

TOP TIP – BEARD-TO-HAIR RATIO

The thing to avoid, especially with a shorter, more cropped (but full) beard, is having your hair the same length as your beard. It creates an unsettling 'which is the top and which is the bottom?' vibe, like that character in *Guess Who?*

 MAINTAINING FACIAL HAIR

As we've mentioned, it's one thing to grow a moustache or a beard, but you have to be prepared to look after it in the same way you would the hair on your head. And, of course, there are easily as many products for you to try. Grooming your beard or moustache is a bit more challenging because the hair tends to be more bristly, but these basic tips will help you avoid a facial-hair fail.

✂ Don't trim too early – whether you're growing a moustache or a beard, the best initial step is to let it grow freely, without trimming, for the first six weeks. As a result, your hair will grow out more fully and evenly (though there will be some variation in length initially).

✂ Wash it like you do your hair – wash it while bathing, but not with a regular shampoo as they often contain agents that remove moisture and natural oils. Consider trying a facial-hair-specific cleanser. Don't be tempted to treat it rough with the towel because it's a bit more robust – go gentle, as you should with your hair, and avoid blow-drying at high temperatures.

✂ Comb and trim to win – perhaps the most important aspect of maintaining your beard or moustache is regular and careful trimming. A moustache comb and/or beard comb or brush is a must, to even out the hair before cutting. Small scissors, for the moustache especially, are vital to trim stray hairs, but the bulk of the work should be done with a trimmer (straightening the 'stache and cropping the bulk of your beard if you have a shorter beard). Fade your neck with your trimmer or shave it – neck beards are a total no.

✂ Condition and style – beard oil/moisturizer conditions and makes the hair less Brillo-pad-like, and moustache wax gives you extra neatness or ridiculous twiddly bits – your call.

CARE AND STYLING PRODUCTS

It's worth taking a closer look at the facial haircare and styling products out there, as there are lots – some more essential than others. The very least you should do for your facial hair is keep it clean and tidy, which involves washing, brushing and trimming. But to take it to the next level and make it appear properly groomed, you need to add in a few more stages.

Facial-hair-specific shampoos and cleansers, used two or three times a week, help to moisturize what is naturally quite wiry and dull hair and are worth investing in. Caring for the skin underneath your facial hair is also important, since it's that much harder to get to. Some might recommend an exfoliating device, but a decent everyday moisturizer, applied as normal, will do most of the work, and when coupled with a lightweight beard balm or beard oil, moisture will be locked in.

When it comes to brushing and combing, you have several options. A moustache comb is typically small in size, with fine teeth, but if your 'stache is particularly bushy you might get away with using the fine end of a beard comb. Beard comb choice depends on the length of your beard – a beard brush will be better for a cropped beard, since the hair needs more persuasion as it's shorter, whereas a larger, wide-toothed wooden comb might be better for a mountain-man style which will need more root-to-tip wrangling. Regular combing will not only help the condition of your beard, by distributing natural oils in the hair, but of course will give it structure and prime it for trimming.

A beard trimmer is an obvious place to start if you're going DIY. The idea is to maintain even length, or shape your beard (you might want shorter sides, to elongate it). This is easier when your beard is short, but less so if you're working with a mass of hair. In which case, you should consider bringing your hairdresser in on the action. Scissors for facial hair, if you're employing a trimmer, are just to catch stray hairs and straighten your moustache. Keeping hair away from your lips and mouth is the best way to avoid trapping food detritus, but if you're washing and combing regularly, you might not care too much.

GO *NATUREL* - BEARD BALM

Grooming products are expensive, so if you can't bring yourself to splash out on something 'just for your facial hair' then why not have a go at making some yourself?

Equipment

Kitchen scales

A small funnel

A pipette

A medium cooking pot (one just for this purpose)

A few candle tins with lids

Ingredients

2oz beeswax

4oz shea butter

7.5 fl oz carrier oil (almond, avocado, coconut, peanut, pomegranate seed, watermelon seed, etc.)

A few drops (small bottle) of essential oil (chamomile, eucalyptus, ginger, lavender, lemon, patchouli, sandalwood, etc.)

Method

Put your pot on a very low heat and add the beeswax. As it begins to melt, add in the shea butter and mix, then add the carrier oil. Stir occasionally to ensure the ingredients are coming together. When the mixture has completely turned to liquid and is mixed, take it off the heat. Immediately add several drops of your selected essential oil and stir well. Next, before the mixture sets, transfer to your candle tins and leave for at least 12 hours to cool and set.

The Rest - of the Body -

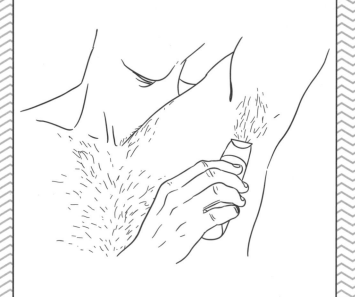

Your head and your face are the most obvious areas to focus your grooming attention, since they're on show most of the time, but of course there are other, less exposed parts of the body to consider. The benefits of grooming your body hair can be numerous – for one, you will be paying close to attention to areas you might not otherwise, so you're more likely to spot anything troubling (like if you wash your car or bike regularly). There's also the bonus of aesthetic appeal – overly hairy bodies are not loved by everyone, especially when it comes to action in the bedroom, so keeping it in check might help there too. The hygienic benefits of removing hair around the pubis (pubic area) and 'sack and crack' area are not evident. It's believed that your pubes reduce friction during sex and trap pheromones, so if you shave them you are inviting cuts and ingrown hairs in very sensitive areas, and if you wax you're losing your bushy buffer. Hair also hides imperfections and softens the lines of less shapely areas of the body (not an issue if you're in shape!). That said, it is a personal choice, and one that many men take.

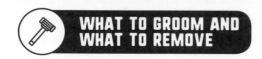

WHAT TO GROOM AND WHAT TO REMOVE

Clearly, there are areas where you will want to eradicate hair, and some where you might just want to keep on top of it:

1. The back – removal is preferable; book yourself in for a waxing.

2. The chest and stomach – use your trimmer; a bit of neat hair is attractive.

3. The arms – upper arms can be waxed, especially if it's sprouting randomly.

4. The armpits – only if this area is excessively, poking-out hairy do you need to trim with scissors.

5. The legs – if it's rampant, trim to take out some of the thickness; otherwise, leave it alone.

6. The backside – a baby-smooth butt is cute; hairy buns are horrid – wax 'em! As for the crack, this area is usually hidden, so the aesthetic value

of hair removal is not obvious. If your sex life involves some action in this area, keeping it bare might be preferable.

7 The genital area (pubis, penis, scrotum) – contentious, as mentioned above, but you are pretty safe with simply trimming your pubis with a guard, to make it look less like a jungle. Wet shaving is possible for the pubis, but it's a sensitive area, so you need to be slow and steady to avoid cuts and rashes – and always follow up with a sensitive post-shave moisturizer, even when using a foil-guard shaver. The same goes for the penis and scrotum. Do bare genitals look porn star or pre-pubescent? That might depend on the size of your enchilada, but ultimately it's your call.

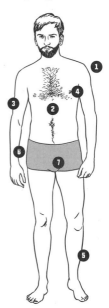

TOP TIP - BODY HAIR

If your body hair is at 'bear level', you might be more inclined to look at in-depth grooming. If you're new to body grooming, and you're only moderately hairy, you might want to focus on the largest and potentially hairiest areas to begin with (chest and back). A word of caution, though: once you start taking hair off your body, you kind of have to keep going indefinitely, which can be something of a chore. It's also important to remember, if your hair is dense and dark, you want to avoid creating harsh lines, which again will mean more work.

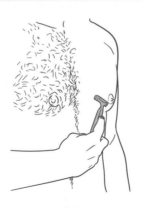

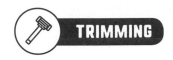

TRIMMING

This is arguably the most common and amenable option when it comes to manscaping, so you'll want to invest in an electric trimmer. There are lots to choose from, but it's generally recommended that you keep your hair/beard trimmer separate from your body grooming trimmer. A body grooming trimmer will have design features that are specific to these areas of the body, such as shorter comb lengths, sensitive-to-skin adaptations like rounded blades, and waterproofing for use in the shower, which might not translate as well for the hair further up. Some more expensive models will feature a clipper and a foil shaver, which means you can crop both long and short hairs with one piece of kit.

DRY TRIMMING

If we're talking about areas with bulk hair – pubis and chest, but not limited to these areas if you're especially hairy – then the best place to start is dry shaving with a trimmer. In these kinds of areas you want to reduce bulk and just make everything look tidy.

You could opt for some body grooming scissors, which have rounded-off ends to avoid any unwanted injuries, which can be useful for flyaways or just as a less intensive overall trim in the longest areas.

WET SHAVING

The obvious option for a wet shave is a cartridge razor (a multi-blade option with some sort of balm or buffer built in would help), but a more popular option, at least for beginners, is a trimmer/shaver. Certain trimmers are designed to function in the shower, which means you can take advantage of the benefits of wet shaving – namely, shaving cream – while you trim your sensitive areas. Here are some tips for when you're going for the wet option:

X If there is a bulk of hair and your aim is to shave it down to nothing, start by dry-trimming the area in question.

X Get your shower going and get in. The heat will cause your hair to swell a little and become easier to shave.

X Next, clean the area to remove dirt and dead skin.

X Use a high-quality, sensitive-skin shaving cream, applied thinly. When your delicate areas are at risk, it's no time to penny-pinch. Your shaving cream not only functions as a lubricant, but it should also help moisturize and soothe. Remember to add more where you need to – don't just settle for one application.

X Shave in all directions. Body hair grows unevenly, at all angles (if you haven't already been grooming), so be sure to make multiple steady passes with your shaver and resist the urge to press too firmly.

X Aftershave care is essential in this situation. Opt for sensitive-skin products with no alcohol.

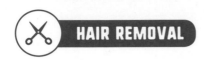

HAIR REMOVAL

If you're after a more long-lasting solution for your body hair, there are plenty of options. You could go DIY and use wax strips. This will last up to six weeks, but it will make your eyes water. Aside from following the instructions on the box carefully, the key is to treat the skin after waxing with a soothing spray or gel, and use a cold, wet cloth to take the initial sting away. If the thought of inflicting pain on yourself puts you off, just book an appointment and have it done by someone else.

TOP TIP - WAX ON, WAX OFF

Before you start, be sure that the area you're waxing is clean and dry. You can also skim over the hair with a trimmer (on a $1/3$ inch setting) to make the waxing easier. Rip in the opposite direction to which the hair is growing and remember to be swift, like Mr Miyagi catching that fly!

Hair removal creams have been popular for many years and make getting rid of unwanted growth easier and less painful. These depilatory creams only take a few minutes to work – they weaken hair at its root and it washes away. They're great for hard-to-reach areas (not your genitals!), but of course the results only last about a week. There's also the chance that you might react adversely to some of the chemicals found in the cream, so it's best to use it on a small patch before covering yourself from head to toe!

The most hi-tech (and expensive) option for long-lasting hair removal is laser treatment. It works on the cells that produce the hair by halting their function and is especially effective on large areas like the back and butt. There are DIY options, but since it involves high-powered beams of cell-destroying light, you might want to leave it to the professionals.

- Skin -

For something that covers you from head to toe and has so many essential functions, a lot of us are guilty of taking our skin for granted. It's a biological wonder, acting as a barrier against infection and capable of repairing itself, and is considered to be an organ in its own right (albeit an external one). But the skin can also be the source of various problems – blemishes, dandruff, rashes – which is all the more reason to get clued up and pay it some close attention. People as far back as the ancient Egyptians realized that keeping your skin in good health was worthwhile, using essential oils as moisturizers. And although historically the focus for skincare has been women, today men are just as likely to get involved.

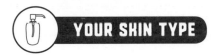

YOUR SKIN TYPE

Just like your hair, your skin has a natural condition which will vary from person to person. This can change through the seasons, but there are generally three accepted 'types' of skin, and this can be good to know if you want to take proper care of it. Your skin type can affect your entire body, but it tends to be most noticeable on the face.

✗ Dry skin – as you might expect, dry skin lacks moisture – or rather the natural oil that keeps skin soft and supple. If you have dry skin, you'll notice tightness (especially in the face) and potential flaking.

✗ Normal/combination skin – people with 'normal' skin type are less likely to experience dry skin breakouts, but it's not out of the question. Generally, though, this skin type is stable and supple without much variation. 'Combination' skin consists of both 'normal' and sometimes 'oily' skin, but again is not seriously prone to breakouts.

✂ Oily skin – of course, oily skin means an excess of oil (sebum) which can clog pores and lead to blemishes, etc. The skin might have a shiny look to it and will be noticeably oily to the touch.

HOW TO DETERMINE YOUR SKIN TYPE

There's a basic way of telling what skin type you have (apart from the more obvious clues). Start by washing with a mild soap or cleanser, rinse with lukewarm water and carefully pat dry. After an hour, if you notice you have oil on your nose, forehead and cheeks, you most likely have oily skin. If there's a little shine on just your nose and forehead, you have normal/combination skin. If there is no shine on your face and if when you pull a few facial expressions it feels tight, you have dry skin.

ETHNICITY AND SKIN TYPE

Ethnicity is also a factor in skin type, in the respect that it can determine how the skin reacts to various environmental conditions. For example, though all skin needs to be protected from the sun, darker skin tones have more natural protection from UV rays (and lighter skin tones have less). Research indicates that darker skin is least likely to be irritated when the skin's natural barrier is compromised – for example, during shaving – whereas Asian skin is most easily irritated. You might already know these things from experience, but it's worth keeping in mind when you're considering how best to look after your skin.

SENSITIVE SKIN

Sensitive skin is not a type, but it's a common occurrence. In fact, skin can become sensitive at any point in your life, for various reasons. Sensitivity comes as a result of an increased susceptibility to allergens, chemicals and bacteria due to the skin's natural barrier being compromised. This can also go hand in hand with dry skin, which when sensitive can be unpredictable – a red or dry patch can emerge seemingly out of nowhere. Sensitive skin is something that has to be managed (rather than 'cured'), but there are lots of simple things you can do to improve the health of your skin (more of which in the following pages).

TOP TIP – MALE SKIN

You might think that skin is skin, but the fact is that male skin differs from female skin. It is 20 per cent thicker, has more collagen, and has more active sebaceous glands, meaning it's more likely to be oily and prone to acne. Consider these factors when choosing skincare products.

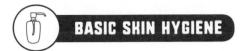

BASIC SKIN HYGIENE

This might sound so obvious that it needn't be covered, but there's more to basic hygiene than you might think when it comes to your skin. We're talking about the first step in the process, which is cleansing your skin of dirt and impurities. And here we need to make an important point – cleansing and caring for your face should differ from cleansing and caring for your body, mainly because the skin acts differently.

For more information about how our lifestyle can affect the health of your skin, turn to p.173.

CLEANSING YOUR FACE

Removing dirt, sweat, oil (sebum) and make-up (if you use it) from your face – all of which might create pore blockages – is the aim, as well as exfoliation (removal of dead skin cells). Ideally, this should happen twice a day, but you'll be able to judge the frequency according to your own skin's condition.

What's wrong with soap and water, you say? Well, nothing, except that you can do so much better nowadays so you'd be silly not to.

There are many cleansing products tailored for men, often with active ingredients to combat typical male issues like dry skin and excess oil. Cream cleansers are, as you might expect, 'creamy', though they are intended to be washed out. They often contain calming, skin-nourishing elements and are suited to be a go-to product for daily use. Oil cleansers are even more rich than cream, and so potentially more nourishing, though they are a little trickier to apply, being more fluid.

You can also find specific cleansers, which focus on one particular aspect of skincare – exfoliation, oil reduction, sensitivity – which will be of benefit if you want to focus on these in particular.

CLEANSING YOUR BODY

The idea is largely the same for the rest of your body – removing dirt and sweat – but of course there's a larger area to focus on and skin tends to be tougher, so you can be more adventurous with things like exfoliation. Here are a few tips:

✂ Take short, tepid showers or baths rather than long, hot ones, which remove too much oil from the skin and dry it out.

✂ Use a gentle cleanser, regardless of your skin type.

✂ Help exfoliation by using a body polisher or loofah (not recommended for sensitive and/or dry skin).

✂ Clean your legs and feet! Don't just accept that they got wet so they're done.

✂ Pat your skin dry, instead of rubbing it vigorously, to retain some moisture and reduce stress.

TO POWDER OR NOT TO POWDER

Talcum powder has for years been used not only for babies but by hygiene-conscious men who want to ensure their nether regions are as fresh and dry as possible. However, recent studies have cast doubt over its safety. According to the American Cancer Society, talc has been connected to an increased risk of cancer, though this was ovarian cancer in women. The ACS says that average body talcum powder, if inhaled, is 'not classifiable as to carcinogenicity in humans'. More research is being done to make the situation clear, but for now, if you use talc on a regular basis, it might be worth reducing your usage.

CARING FOR YOUR SKIN

Once you have your cleansing down, you should consider investing in a product or two to help condition and tone your skin. As we mentioned above, men's skin naturally has more collagen in it, so it will have a firmer appearance. But don't get too excited. Signs of ageing appear much more abruptly in men, and wrinkles are very pronounced. So it's a good idea to put the extra work in, while you're still looking good. Plus, you'll get a buzz from feeling like your skin is in top condition.

MOISTURIZERS

As with cleansing, there are different products for different areas – face, body, hands (but there are also combo creams) – and, of course, your skin type will determine which is the best one for you. It's about balance once again – you don't want to use an oily product if you have oily skin, etc.

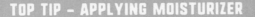

TOP TIP - APPLYING MOISTURIZER

Apply moisturizer as soon as you're done washing, while your skin is damp (pat yourself over with a towel so you're not sodden). It's much more effective than applying to dry skin. Scoop or squeeze out a small amount of moisturizer onto your fingers and dab it evenly onto the area you're aiming to cover. Rub it in carefully. If you're planning on using any sort of make-up (see p.91), allow the moisturizer to dry before applying.

Face

Let's start at the top. Your face is the centre of attention most of the time, and there is a vast choice of moisturizer available, but if you stick to the principle of balance you won't go too far wrong. The table opposite gives you an outline of what to go for (and what to avoid) according to skin type.

SKIN TYPE/ CONDITION	GO FOR	AVOID
Dry skin	Products that are 'rich' but 'non-greasy'; 'exfoliating'; containing shea butter	Products with alcohol or its derivatives or acidic ingredients (citrus, mint) that will remove oil; products that mention 'toning' which will tighten your skin further
Normal/ combination skin	Products that are 'lightweight' and 'oil-free'; 'gel' (as opposed to 'cream'); 'hydrating' and 'toning'	Products described as 'for dry skin'
Oily	'Gel' (as opposed to 'cream'); products described as 'oil-free', 'no-shine' and 'cleansing'	Products described as 'for dry skin'
Sensitive	'Calming' and 'soothing' 'cream' (as opposed to gel, although gels with aloe vera are good); products that are 'hypoallergenic' and 'scent-free'	'Revitalizing' and 'exfoliating'; products with alcohol or its derivatives or acidic ingredients (citrus, mint)

GO *NATUREL* – NATURAL MOISTURIZERS

There are many natural products which have benefits for your skin simply as they are. So if you're struggling to find a product that you're happy with, or if you just want to avoid man-made ingredients, why not try applying some **coconut oil** (which you can also use for cooking) straight from the pot, heating it up in your palms first. Or try some classic **cucumber**, which can be pureed and mixed with a few drops of honey to make a cooling mask suitable for all skin types. The one most people know about is **aloe vera**. You can literally pick a leaf of this succulent, break it in half and apply the gel that you will see glistening on the inner flesh of the leaf – it doesn't get much more natural than that!

EXFOLIATORS

Removing dead skin cells through exfoliation is a worthwhile step in any skincare routine. Your skin is constantly renewing itself, and in this process dead skin cells gather at the surface, forming what is known as the *stratum corneum*. These dead cells fall away naturally (though they are so small you can't see them) but when they don't fall away of their own accord, they can combine with the skin's natural oil and clog your pores – which means spots. So it's a good idea to help them on their way by exfoliating regularly, which can be done by using tools like a body polisher or a loufah (this is not recommended for your face, especially if you have dry/sensitive skin) and/or an exfoliating, oil-free cleanser. This will also make your skin look healthier, giving it a radiant glow.

Exfoliating products often contain granules of some sort – salt, sugar or other natural particles – which help loosen and remove dead skin cells. Again, these can be irritating to sensitive skin, so avoid them if that's you. You should also avoid products with 'microbeads' which have been proven to be harmful to the environment (and which many countries have now banned).

DANGER ZONES

Dramatic heading aside, we're talking about the areas that might need some special attention (and maybe some special products). As we've mentioned already, there are slight differences to the condition and function of skin in different places – some areas get more wear and tear, some are naturally more sensitive, etc. Here's a list of some common hotspots and how to look after them:

✂ Face – we've already covered this quite a bit (see p.41), but it's worth mentioning that, as a result of shaving, men's faces are subject to an increased level of stress. Shaving can help to exfoliate, but in doing so it can also go too deep into the *stratum corneum*, which lets out moisture and causes dry skin. A gentle shaving cream/gel and an appropriate aftershave balm or lotion (but not aftershave itself, as it's alcohol-based) will help.

✂ Hands – your hands are always moving and touching things, which means they are exposed to the highest numbers of potential contaminants, and the skin is being physically stressed in various ways. On top of this, cheaper handwash (often containing oil-stripping alcohol) will dry them out, so it's a good idea to keep them supple with a non-greasy moisturizer. (Now you know why your grandma has that hand lotion next to the soap!)

✂ Elbows – how many times have you looked at your elbows? Probably never! Which means you might not have noticed how dry they are. Elbows are another hard-wear point for skin and as such it's often tough and dry. Not so significant in the winter, but when summer comes and your guns are on display, you don't want to look like a tortoise. Apply body lotion regularly.

✂ Feet/soles/heels – another often-neglected area is the feet. We've already mentioned giving them attention in the shower, which will help with exfoliation, but your feet are one of the thickest, toughest, and most-used areas of skin on your body and therefore prone to dryness and cracking. Keep this at bay by regular exfoliation – there are plenty of tools, such as pedicure files and pumice stones, to remove hard skin, which are often most effective after you've soaked your feet in Epsom salts or another effective skin softener.

CARE THROUGH THE SEASONS

Even if our skincare game is on lock, it pays to be aware of the particular challenges the changing of the seasons might pose.

WEATHER	CHALLENGE TO SKIN	HOW TO HELP
Warm	Increased oil production (face)	Use a cleanser/toner/ moisturizer for oily skin
Strong sun	UV exposure (all areas)	Wear sunscreen (in accordance with your natural tolerance); cover up more (with a tasteful hat, stylish shirt, etc.); keep hydrated
Windy	Skin drying out (exposed areas)	Take a travel-size moisturizer out with you or, if you'd rather not do that, be sure to moisturize well when indoors. Keeping something at work is always a winner.
Cold	Skin drying out (exposed areas); skin cracking (lips and hands)	Stop skin drying out in general by upping your moisturizer application and covering up as much as you can. Protect your lips with a balm and your hands with an intensive, winter moisturizer.

BLEMISHES AND IMPERFECTIONS

It's all good if your skincare routine is working wonders for you, but what about when, despite your efforts, your skin throws you a curveball and you end up with imperfections – be it spots (acne), dry patches (*xerosis*), or rashes (inflammation/dermatitis). Here we'll cover some of the most common issues, as well as some of the more persistent ones like eczema, psoriasis and rosacea. It's important to note that the best course of action, in the case of a persistent problem, is to consult your doctor.

ACNE

Nearly everyone will have experienced pimples as a teenager, mostly as a result of a hormonal surge, but they can come back to haunt you in adult life. It's all down to your hair follicles getting blocked by excess oil (sebum) that has mixed with dead skin cells (like we mentioned in the previous section on exfoliators). So, for the most part, preventing acne is as simple as doing a good job cleansing and/or exfoliating. It can also be caused by stress, which is helped by regular exercise, among other things; heavy sweating, which you can take care of after your exercise by cleansing; and environmental factors like humidity, which you can counter by pre-emptive cleansing.

If your acne is persistent or extensive, it's advisable to visit your pharmacist or doctor for advice.

DRY SKIN

We've already talked about dry skin as a skin type, but you might encounter it as a one-off, seemingly random occurrence, medically termed *xerosis*. It can be caused by environmental factors, as discussed, but it can also be triggered by spending too long in a hot shower or bath (so cut down your time in the bath/shower and use tepid water), using a harsh, oil-stripping soap (use a gentle option, usually 'fragrance-free', and pat skin dry) or wearing skin-irritating clothing, like wool (wear cotton for the time being).

More long-term skin conditions are covered later on pp.184–189.

RASHES

'Rash' is not a medical term and can refer to any number of skin conditions that appear inflamed or irritated. A common 'rash' is contact dermatitis, which is essentially when skin becomes temporarily inflamed as a result of contact with an irritant. The irritant could be a man-made chemical, like solvents, oils and detergents, or an ingredient in your soap, styling product or moisturizer. Try to narrow down the culprit, reduce your exposure and treat with an emollient in the meantime.

And then there's 'razor burn' – redness, burning, itchiness and possibly small bumps on the skin. This is essentially caused by the skin and hair follicles being irritated by the scraping razor. So, in some ways, it's inherent to wet shaving, but there are lots of things you can do to avoid or minimize it:

✄ Clean and exfoliate the skin before shaving.

✄ Heat the area to be shaved with a hot towel to soften the hair.

✂ Use a mild shaving cream, regardless of your skin type, and don't shave an area without a covering of cream.

✂ Always use a sharp razor (no more than five shaves old).

✂ Use short, light strokes and shave with the grain of your hair.

✂ Use cold water to close your pores off when you're done.

✂ Pat your skin dry with a towel.

✂ Apply a sensitive post-shave balm to soothe the skin.

RAZOR BUMPS

Razor bumps (*pseudofolliculitis barbae*) are a delayed effect of shaving, as opposed to razor burn, which will be noticeable very soon after. They occur when a hair follicle that has been skewed by shaving grows back underneath the skin and causes a tiny abscess. They can be prevented by following the same steps listed above.

ECZEMA

Aside from short-term irritations and blemishes, there are a number of conditions that can be more long-term. Eczema is one of the most common, though it is not a lifelong ('chronic') condition but one that can both worsen or improve with time. It appears as widespread red, cracked, itchy blotches which can 'flare up' at different times and as a result of different irritants. Aside from the physical annoyance, it can be a source of anxiety for men who are trying to look and feel their best.

There is no one cause – many people who suffer from common allergies are prone to it – but the same things that irritate dry skin (see p.65) can make eczema worse. It is not contagious.

Eczema can respond well to a basic moisturizer,

though often it requires prescribed corticosteroids to be properly calmed. Controlling your eczema can also be about learning what might be triggering it – heat, detergents, certain foods. If you think you might have eczema, consult your doctor who will offer advice on how to recognize your triggers and manage the condition in the meantime.

PSORIASIS

Psoriasis has some things in common with eczema, in that it produces non-contagious widespread red, cracked, itchy patches, but they tend to be covered by thicker, scalier skin. It's also arguably less temperamental, not so affected by environmental factors, but can appear out of nowhere. Unlike eczema it is a chronic hereditary condition resulting from a flaw in the autoimmune system which causes dead skin to build up on the surface much quicker than it would normally. There are a number of psoriasis-specific products out there – like tar-based shampoo for the scalp and oil-based emollients for the skin

– but the most effective treatments are obtained by prescription or professional consultation.

ROSACEA

Rosacea is another common skin complaint that is characterized by long-lasting redness in the face, which may also involve increased visibility of blood vessels and a stinging sensation. Like eczema it can be temperamental, and when present it can be embarrassing, as it has quite a dramatic effect on the face. Factors such as sunlight, stress, certain foods (alcohol and spicy food) and cold weather can trigger rosacea, so paying attention to these things can stop it getting worse. Sensitive-skin cleansers and moisturizers are recommended, as is regular sun protection, even on overcast days. Electric shavers are recommended over razors.

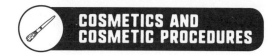

COSMETICS AND COSMETIC PROCEDURES

There might be times when all of your skincare dedication falls short, and no matter what you reasonably do to keep yourself looking good, you can't overcome that acne or those wrinkles. Aside from improving your overall health and well-being (see Section 5), there are both short-term methods for cheating your way through, or long-term methods for resolving the issues.

COSMETICS

Make-up lines for men are (in 2018) still a relatively new thing. That's not to say that men haven't been using make-up for decades (millennia, if you count the ancient Egyptians and Sumerians), but products aimed at what manufacturers *think* men want – for example, YSL's Touche Éclat concealer for men is unfragranced and more matte – are now hitting the mainstream.

How people use make-up is a personal choice, but often it can come down to either applying it to conceal (e.g. hiding an imperfection with concealer) or to reveal (e.g. showing off, enhancing or drawing attention to a particular feature – using eyeshadow or colored nail varnish) – or both. For the purposes of this book, we'll stick to the less showy use of make-up, as grooming is arguably more about maintenance than it is about being glamorous.

TOP TIP – SKIN TYPE AND TONE

With make-up, considering your skin type is key. You will find products that are suitable for dry, oily and normal/combination skin types. Finding make-up to match your skin tone is a bit more complicated than reading the label. You can get an idea of your skin's 'undertone' by looking at the veins in your wrists. If they are a greenish, yellowish color you

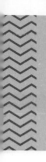

have warm undertones; if they are more purplish or bluish, you have cool undertones; if they are a mix of these colors, you have neutral undertones. This will give you a steer on what range of tones you should look for.

So what kinds of make-up could be go-to options for the well-groomed guy? Here's a list of items you might want to consider (and what they do):

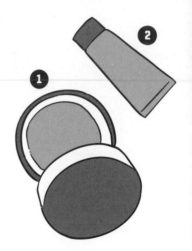

1. Anti-shine powder – as you might guess, this is aimed at people with oily skin. It often comes as a powder, so applying with a brush is recommended, and will give a matte look.

2. Concealer – no prizes for guessing what this one does! When matched properly with your skin tone this semi-solid cream will help to hide blemishes. It is often used for smaller areas. If you want to mask redness, a green concealer (made in the color green, which will neutralize any strong tone) is invaluable.

3 Foundation – this will provide an all-over, smooth finish to your face. It might be liquid (apply with a finger) or powder (apply with a brush).

4 Brow powder – match to your hair color and you're good to go. You'll need a finer brush if you want to use this on your brows, but it's also effective to fill in any patchy parts of your beard.

5 Bronzer – often comes as a powder and, as its name suggests, the idea is to create a bronzed look to the face. A 'bronzer brush' will be the best way to apply a powder, but it also comes as a cream.

COSMETIC PROCEDURES

There could be any number of reasons you might consider a paid-for, professional cosmetic procedure – from a simple spray tan to get into the holiday swing, to removing an embarrassing tattoo or having surgery on a feature that you are unhappy with. Here's a list of the most common procedures and what you might expect (for all of these, you should consult a relevant professional before you go through with it):

✂ Spray tan – exposure to UV causes all sorts of issues for skin, so fake tan has come into its own. Tanning solution is sprayed onto your body and reacts with the uppermost layer of skin cells, turning them a darker shade. There are oil- and water-based solutions, and if you have sensitive skin you should go for the latter. The tan can last up to ten days if you moisturize every day and keep the dyed skin from shedding.

✂ Laser tattoo removal – there could be any number of reasons why you might want to get a tattoo removed (and we won't go into them here – your regrets are your own!) but the good news is that it is possible to have them removed. The bad news is that it's not guaranteed to remove the tat completely, it's likely to take several sessions (six to ten) and there are a number of unwelcome after-effects such as blisters, swelling, bleeding, a ghost image, permanent scarring and hyperpigmentation. There is a higher risk of hyperpigmentation for guys with darker skin tones. Of course, you should start with a consultation and plenty of research before you go down this route.

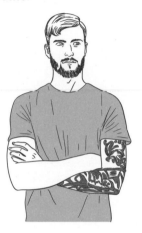

✂ 'Bro-tox' – the attraction of Botox (*Botulinum toxin* injections) is understandable, especially if you're bothered by creeping signs of ageing in your face. Facial lines and wrinkles are made less obvious with this treatment, but at $200–$450 (in 2018) per session it doesn't come cheap. There is also the fact that it might not result in the desired effect, it's not permanent (lasts around six months), you could experience headaches, bruising and facial droopiness after the injections, and signs of ageing will still be present in areas you can't treat. If that doesn't put you off, you should do your utmost to find a reputable practitioner and have a face-to-face meeting.

X Dermal fillers – like Botox, this treatment is an injection of a substance into the face to lessen the appearance of lines and wrinkles and plump up areas you want plumping – collagen is a common dermal filler. They are similar in price to Botox and basically the same drawbacks apply.

X Microdermabrasion – this is a more intensive, mechanical version of your regular exfoliation, removing dead skin cells and encouraging new ones to be produced as well as increasing the elasticity and clarity of your skin and softening fine age lines. It can be used all over the body, but the face is an obvious area, since it's on show a bit more. After-effects include slight tenderness and redness, but there is the less intensive try-at-home option of a microdermabrasion cloth.

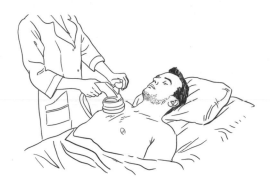

✂ Hyperpigmentation removal – hyperpigmentation (darker areas on your skin caused by excess melanin production) can occur as the result of skin trauma, as mentioned above with tattoo removal, but also as a result of a skin disorder or ageing in general. In this treatment, lasers can help to boost collagen production and lessen the appearance of the pigmentation. Blistering and burning is a risk with this treatment, as is damage to the eyes if the lasers are used improperly. Plus you will require multiple sessions.

COSMETIC SURGERY

We said at the start of this chapter that grooming is essentially about maintenance and healthy habits. All of the above push the boundary of this credo, and so in some ways are things to look at if grooming isn't working for you, and this goes even more so for surgery. However, more and more men are opting for things like blepharoplasty (eyelid lift), rhinoplasty (nose re-shaping) and gynecomastia (moob reduction). It's a potentially life-changing route, though costly and not without serious risks, so it will require serious thought and thorough consultation with a surgeon.

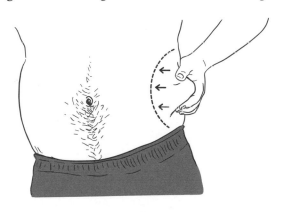

- Nails -

If you've ever stubbed your toe or shut your finger in a door, you'll know that the ends of your fingers and toes are pretty damn sensitive. This is an advantage for all sorts of reasons – your sense of touch for one – but it's also a drawback when injury is concerned. Your nails help to protect the soft tissue at the ends of these digits and help you to use your fingers like a pincer for accurate grip.

In terms of grooming, there are some essential ways to keep them in good shape (for them to function, not cause problems and not gross people out) and additional ways to keep them looking extra healthy.

- Fingers -

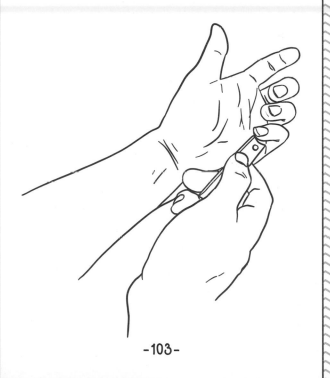

BASIC HYGIENE AND MAINTENANCE

As we mentioned in the Skin section, your hands are one of the more hard-working parts of your body, so they deserve some care. They are also often focal points when interacting with other people, since they're moving about and catching the eye. If your hands – and nails – look like they belong to a werewolf's stunt double, you're going to make a bad impression, not to mention invite all sorts of hygiene issues. Here's a guide to keeping your nails in good shape.

TOP TIP – INVEST IN A NAIL KIT

First things first – get yourself a quality nail care kit, consisting of at least a pair of nail scissors and a nail file (emery board). There is also a good argument to have separate finger and nail tools, as described below. High-quality, hand-finished steel tools are the best.

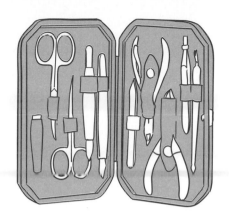

Trimming

How long is too long? Well, it's a personal choice, of course, but you're inviting all sorts of dirt and grime to become lodged underneath if you let your nails get much longer than the end of your finger. As a rule of thumb (and finger!), if you can feel your nail when you touch the end of your finger, it's time to trim.

There is a strong argument for not using clippers at all for trimming your fingernails. The average pair of fingernail clippers (the smaller ones, about ⅓ inch in width, as opposed to the larger ones which are for your toes) is a bit of a crude instrument – they're made from soft steel and lose their edge very quickly, and so will not be cutting properly. Even the lever concept itself is flawed, since they're often fussy to use, meaning you make a mess of the cut and end up with jagged, damaged nails which will catch and grow back unevenly.

Whatever you're using, make sure your tool has been washed out and dried first (as if you don't already know, the stuff that lurks underneath your nails can be dirty and smelly). With scissors in hand, consider how much you should take off and how to approach the cutting. You should aim to leave a tiny bit of white at the end, which means you're not cutting the nail back beyond the natural bed. (You can see the bed if you cut too much off, it's a recess with a natural edge to it.) You should trim an arc that mirrors the (inverted) shape of your proximal fold, which is the point at which the skin ends and the nail begins. Whether using scissors or clippers, work your way around the arc in a series of cuts. Try not to trim off the sides of your nails as cutting too close can lead to ingrown nails; leave the corners square and break out the emery file.

Filing

Now it's time to take the corners off your trimmed nails and smooth any slightly rough edges. The trick is not to saw back and forth, but use a gentle, one-way motion, filing at a slight angle from below the nail. If that all seems a bit much, think about it like this: if someone was being affectionate by holding your hand, stroking your neck, or something more intimate, would you want to feel the scrape of a sharp nail?

Cuticle care

A cuticle is a dead layer of skin that occurs just beyond the point where your finger skin ends and your nail begins. It looks like a 'ghost' layer of nail, as if a very thin layer of clear varnish has dried in a jagged line near the beginning of your nail. It should not be confused with your proximal nail fold, which is the seal that is present between where your skin ends and your nail begins. This seal is there to keep out germs, so if disturbed – some salons insist on cutting it, which is not advisable – it can invite infection.

Excess cuticle can lead to hangnails (those annoying breakaway bits of nail that can occur at the start of your nail or on the sides), which can be painful and become infected, so the idea is to reduce the cuticle layer. This can be done by 'pushing back' the cuticle layer with a tool so it doesn't intrude onto the nail itself. This is arguably best left to a professional, since the nearby proximal nail fold is so important. A gentler alternative is to exfoliate your cuticles by rubbing them with a towel directly after showering – or using a soft nail brush – and by applying some cuticle oil or hand moisturizer to keep them hydrated. If you do decide to get a professional manicure, be sure to ask for your cuticles to be 'pushed back' not 'cut'.

SPECIAL TREATMENTS – MANICURE

If you're going the extra mile with your nail care at home, you might be happy with how your fingernails are looking and feeling. But there's no substitute for some professional attention now and

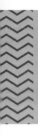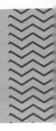

again. With a manicure, aside from having your nails tended to by an expert, the experience can be supremely relaxing and might well involve a hand massage of some kind.

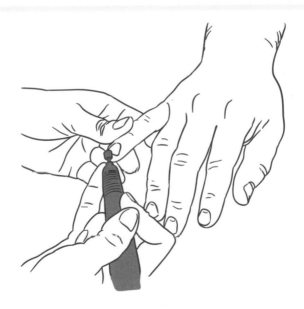

COMMON FINGERNAIL PROBLEMS

We've looked at how to take basic care of your nails, but if, despite your best efforts, you have issues, here's some help.

✂ Ingrown nail – when your nail is growing into the surrounding skin, causing pain and possible infection. If you trim a nail at the very sides, encouraging it to grow where it shouldn't, or leave a sharp corner, or tend to bite your nails, you're asking for an ingrown nail. If your finger is swollen or you suspect it's infected, see your doctor. If it seems more minor, soak your finger in warm water a few times a day, drying well afterwards, to reduce irritation.

✂ Ridged nail – you might notice horizontal ridges in your nails, which make them look uneven. These occur when the natural production of the nail is interrupted, often by trauma to the nail. Aside from making your nail look a bit rough and misshapen, these ridges are harmless and will grow out. If they don't, see your doctor.

✂ Split nail – these are vertical (and sometimes horizontal) splits in the nail which give them a jagged, flaky look with uneven layers developing on top of one another. Brittle nail syndrome is one cause, but often it's a result of working with water, with regular wetting and drying of the hands. Wearing gloves is an obvious step to keep this at bay, along with keeping your nails well-trimmed and healthy by applying an all-purpose skin or hand-specific moisturizer.

✂ Infected nail – any serious infection, such as severe redness, swelling or discoloration, should be treated by a health professional.

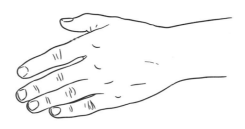

- Toes -

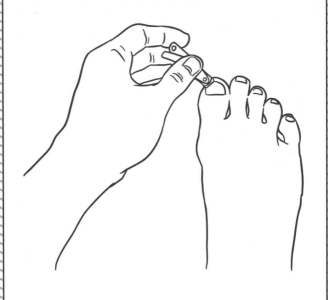

We mentioned earlier that your hands get quite a lot of stick since they're used so much – well, the same goes for your feet, except that you can hide your sins more easily as, unless the weather's nice, they're covered up! That is, until it's time for bed and your partner reels in terror at the sight of your manky, misshapen man-hooves. But don't worry, this section will put you on the right path.

BASIC HYGIENE AND MAINTENANCE

Precisely because they are hidden – stuffed into shoes, collecting sweat, being abused through sport and other activities – is why you need to give your toes more attention.

Trimming

If you've read the advice about fingernails (pp.103–111), you've pretty much got yourself covered. However, there are a few important differences which are worth going over. Firstly, you shouldn't use the same tool to cut your fingernails as you do for your toenails. There's a basic hygiene principle behind this, which is to say that you don't want to transmit anything from your feet (sweatier, washed fewer times, more bacteria-prone) to your fingers and so to your mouth. Even if you're washing and drying your tools, you might not cleanse them completely, or you might just forget to do it. So make it easy for yourself.

Secondly, chances are your fingernail tool won't be sufficient for your toenails. If you have a nice small pair of scissors for your fingernails, they might buckle under the pressure of trimming your toenails, which are much thicker – especially the big toe! So consider investing in a pair of toenail pliers (not levered clippers, which, as we've discussed, have some major drawbacks). These bad boys will make short work of even the toughest nails.

Filing

As with your fingernails, you should use an emery file to take off any rough edges and to smooth the corners that are left after cutting. It's especially important not to trim the sides of your toenails as they are more prone to ingrowing. Your feet are under a lot of pressure as you walk, which means any jagged bit of nail will be biting into your skin all the more. Multiply this effect if you're a keen runner. So, even if you skip this stage for your fingers, don't skip it for your toes.

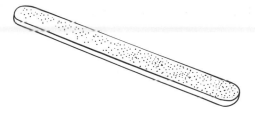

Cuticle care

As valuable for your toenails as it is for your fingernails. Hangnails are especially painful on your toes, which you'll know if you've ever tried walking around with one that has become inflamed. And they can catch on your socks as you put them on, which is so damn annoying.

SPECIAL TREATMENTS – PEDICURE

Just like a manicure, pedicures can be a joyful, relaxing treat. And once again you'll have the option of additional care beyond your toenails, such as dead skin removal and a massage, making it a worthwhile trip (as long as you're not too ticklish!).

COMMON TOENAIL PROBLEMS

1. Ingrown nails – as mentioned above, arguably more common for toenails than for fingernails. Consult your doctor if your condition persists.

2. Thickened nails – often the result of trauma to the nail bed, like if you drop something on your toe. It can also mean the nail grows unevenly. A podiatrist will be able to thin the nail for you, if you want to restore the natural look for cosmetic reasons.

3. Fungal infection – this unfortunate condition is displeasing to the eye as it results in a thickened, discolored nail which might also separate from the nail bed. You can treat the infection with an anti-fungal medicine from your pharmacy, and a podiatrist can help with the trimming and rejuvenation of the nail. If you have a persistent problem, consult your doctor.

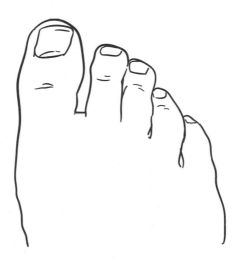

Mouth and Ears

A 'Hollywood smile' is something you might have heard mentioned before – it's supposed to denote a flawless set of pearly-white teeth and immaculate gums – but, given the reputation of this cosmetic-obsessed area of LA, you might be forgiven for thinking it just means 'fake'. Indeed, modern dentistry in general has come a long way since it was established by French surgeon Pierre Fauchard in the eighteenth century and is as much about cosmetic appeal as it is about proper function. But there's also a lot more you can do at home now, so much so that a visit to the dentist might only consist of a 10-minute check-up once a year.

And what good is a perfect smile without clean ears to receive all of those loving compliments? Ears are arguably less glamorous, but should have a significant place in any man's grooming regime. This section will cover all of the essentials for these two areas.

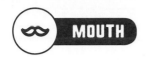

MOUTH

Your mouth sees a lot of action through the course of an average day – food and drink pass through it, and even in between those times there's activity, including while you're asleep, when you speak and when you breathe. So it goes without saying that it needs special care. Hopefully you were taught this at an early age, but being the well-groomed man you are, you should know that there's more to mouth care than brushing and flossing twice a day.

BASIC HYGIENE

Teeth, gums and tongue

There are lots of things you can do for oral hygiene before you even get near your bathroom cabinet (check out the section on Food and Drink, pp.142–155, for more), but we'll start with the common ways of keeping your mouth in good shape after you've eaten.

✂ Toothpaste – are you getting the best from yours? If your mouth is healthy then you might be able to say 'yes', with confidence, but if you have lingering plaque or bad breath you might benefit from trying a different toothpaste. It's all about selecting one that has the right kind of added extras (as all of them, one would hope, are good at cleaning your teeth). There are toothpastes formulated to help with sensitivity in gums and teeth, to help with whitening, to help combat gingivitis (these might be prescription-only) and added-fluoride toothpastes. Your dentist can advise you on products that might help with these more specific issues, but you can also think about your toothpaste on the basis of how it feels. Does it burn when you use it? Maybe it's too harsh for you, despite its promises of better teeth. Does it leave you feeling a bit sensitive? Whitening toothpastes usually contain abrasive particles, which can actually work to damage your enamel, so use with caution.

✂ Electric vs manual toothbrushes – if you're happy with your toothpaste, you should consider the suitability of your brush. It's widely accepted across the dental profession that electric toothbrushes are more effective at cleaning teeth than manual ones. Soft bristles are recommended for adults, unless you have a gum issue.

TOP TIP – REPLACE YOUR BRUSH AND KEEP IT CLEAN

It's advised that you should change your toothbrush – or brush head, if you're using an electric toothbrush – every three months. To keep the bristles clean, simply rinse, shake off excess water and prop up so it can air dry. Keeping it in a case might feel like you're protecting it, but it actually promotes the growth of bacteria.

✂ Brushing frequency and technique – you might already know that dentists advise that you should brush twice a day. Well, the reality is that once a day might well be enough – if you do it properly! The bacteria which can colonize the nooks and crannies of your mouth take 48 hours to establish themselves enough to cause any damage, so in theory one brushing a day is enough to dislodge them. The benefit of brushing twice, especially before bed, is that you cleanse the mouth of a hard day's work and thus reduce the risk of any build-ups – and if your technique isn't perfect, you're making up for it with round two. An electric brush does the hard work for you, in terms of technique, but if you're still going manual you should aim to replicate what an electric does – multiple short, light strokes (horizontal and vertical), with the brush angled slightly towards your gums.

✂ Flossing – you might also already know that flossing is good for your mouth too. Well, maybe. In 2016 Professor Damien Walmsley, the British Dental Association's scientific adviser, said that 'floss is of little value unless the spaces between your teeth are too tight for the inter-dental brushes to fit without hurting or causing harm.' So, rather than breaking out the floss, consider trying a fuzzy little interdental brush, which will help dislodge food and plaque from between teeth.

✂ Mouthwash – this can be a nice back-up to your brushing routine, but you shouldn't be using it right after you've brushed. This will actually wash away the fluoride that's built up in your mouth during brushing, so it will be having the opposite effect for which it was intended. So, if you're keen to use mouthwash, try using it after lunch (you can pick up a mini-size bottle to keep at work) or after dinner if you brush once in the morning. Either way, you might want to go for an alcohol-free mouthwash, which will be less 'burny'. You should aim to use the mouthwash no more than twice a day.

✂ Tongue scraping – you should always give your tongue a light once-over at the end of a brushing session, but if you feel like that's not enough – especially if your breath is still a bit whiffy – you should consider a tongue scraper. These often look a bit like bubble wands, with a 'loop' of soft plastic at one end which helps lift off odor-causing bacteria from the tongue. That's not to say that bacteria on the tongue is bad (it's a natural part of a healthy mouth), just that an excess may lead to bad breath and a scraper can help out.

✂ Plaque scraping (dental picks) – if you're avid about your dental hygiene then you might have been tempted to purchase a dental pick for home use. This is pretty much the same as what a dentist will use – a narrow, hook-type implement for cleaning between teeth and scraping plaque. Seems like a useful tool, but if you're thinking about using one it's best to confer with your dentist beforehand. If used improperly, a dental pick can damage your teeth's enamel, which is never good.

Lips

We've already talked about taking care of your lips by moisturizing, especially in winter, but you can do a little more. Yes, your lips are flexible, but they too can benefit from exfoliation. There are a number of products you can use, such as a lip scrub, but you can also use your humble toothbrush to do the same job. However – don't use it when it's full of toothpaste! A lot of pastes contain sodium laurel sulphate, which will dry your lips out. Use a clean, slightly wet brush and lightly massage your lips in a circular motion. You'll have softer, more kissable lips in no time!

Breath

If you're doing all of the above and you still seem to suffer from a touch of bad breath, consider your diet. Strong-flavored foods will obviously have an effect, as will things like coffee, beer and wine. If you're dieting and your body is breaking down fat, this can also create a funny smell on your breath.

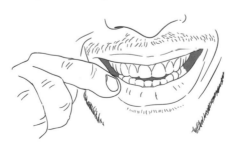

GO *NATUREL* – FRESHEN YOUR BREATH

If you want some simple, natural ways to help keep your breath fresh, check out some of these ideas:

- ✗ **Drink water** – literally washes away odor-causing food and bacteria.

- ✗ **Try green tea** – this contains polyphenols which fight mouth odor.

- ✗ **Eat an apple** – it will neutralize any smells, thanks to the polyphenols it contains.

- ✗ **Baking soda** – mix a teaspoon in a glass of water (and add a drop of peppermint oil), rinse it around your mouth and spit it out like a mouthwash.

- ✗ **Lemon** – cut a wedge, sprinkle a little salt on it and munch it like you would if you were doing a tequila shot. You'll have fresh breath, but you might also have watery eyes! (Be aware that too much citric acid is not good for the enamel on your teeth, so this method should be used sparingly.)

SPECIAL TREATMENTS

When it comes to cosmetic procedures for your teeth, the majority involve expensive dental work. These are things to look into and discuss with your dentist if you're unhappy with the way your teeth look (or if they're deemed necessary by your dentist, for health reasons). We'll take a look at some of the more common ones to give you an idea of what's possible.

✂ Whitening – this involves teeth being bleached to achieve a whiter color. With age and food and drink (and other things, such as smoking), teeth can get darker and dirtier-looking, so the desire to restore them to their former glory is understandable. Your dentist will place gum guards in your mouth and safely apply a substance usually containing hydrogen peroxide to your teeth. There is also such a thing as laser whitening, which (no prizes) uses heat from a laser to enhance the effect of the bleach. This is likely to be very expensive, though, so perhaps not an option for everyone. Minor, temporary side-effects of the procedure might include teeth being more sensitive to cold, and a sore throat and gums. (More about home whitening below.)

✂ Veneers – these are custom-made ceramic coverings that resemble natural teeth, used to create a literal veneer over the front of an unsightly tooth. This procedure is costly and, although it is possible to have the work done independently, it is not recommended unless prescribed by a dentist.

✂ Implants – used to replace missing teeth. A crown is screwed directly into the jaw and is completely secure. The bonus is that often they are indistinguishable from the rest of your teeth and more stable than a denture. However, the treatment can take several months and – you guessed it – it's expensive.

✂ Composite bonding – this is the dental equivalent of using filler to mask and repair cracks. The finished effect has the natural color of your existing teeth and it's one of the least expensive options for repairing and improving the appearance of damaged teeth.

DIY AND NON-SURGICAL OPTIONS

✂ Dental hygienist – aside from a check-up with your dentist, who will really just look for any major issues with your teeth, you should consider seeing a dental hygienist at least once a year. The hygienist will give your teeth a thorough clean (especially good if you have a build-up of plaque, for instance) and also advise you on how best to look after your teeth. It's a little more expensive than your average dentist check-up, but worth it.

✂ Home whitening – aside from paying your dentist to whiten your teeth, there are a number of try-at-home options, which you might find more economical. A typical option is a tray-based whitening kit (trays being the gumshield you fill with the whitening agent and slip over your teeth), which might also include a whitening toothpaste and tooth-polisher to help the process along. Charcoal toothpaste is something that can be used with ease to achieve a more sparkling smile, but perhaps sparingly if it contains heavy abrasive elements. All of the above can be very budget-friendly, so worth a try before paying a visit to the dentist.

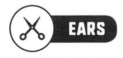

BASIC HYGIENE

We've already covered how to take care of the outside of your ears (see p.45), but what about the inside? Well, the truth is that your ear canal shouldn't need that much attention. Like most things going on inside your body, it's pretty much self-controlling and any interference usually hinders rather than helps. That said, the ears can be a common source of discomfort when issues do occur – and there are steps you can take if your wax does get out of control.

Earwax is not a waste product but actually functions to protect the skin in the ear canal and to stop various bacteria and other foreign objects from entering the sensitive inner ear. As such it doesn't need to be cleansed – in fact, doing so will be taking protection away from your ear. You might have noticed, however, that wax can gather at the opening of your ear and, well, it looks kind of gross! Some people naturally have more wax, some people will create a build-up as a result of having things sit in their ears, like earplugs and hearing aids, and some people might have hairy or narrow ear canals which can lead to an excess.

To clean away the most prominent wax, you should simply use a tissue or a soft cloth to wipe the outer part of your ear – by no means should you dig down into your ear canal with your finger, a twisted up bit of tissue or a dreaded cotton bud! These things will only serve to push wax down further and ultimately cause a blockage or build-up. It can also cause damage to the ear, which you definitely don't want. Ear candles, another commonly touted method, have no proven benefits for wax removal.

GO *NATUREL* - EAR OIL

If you've noticed that there's an excess of earwax present in your outer ear (or if you feel as if it might be blocking your ear) there's a simple, natural remedy you can try before heading to the pharmacy. With your head tilted, simply add a few drops of almond or olive oil to your ear (a pipette will help with this, but if you can't get one use a teaspoon with a little bit of oil on the end). Add the drops for a few days in a row. You may feel the wax soften and disperse inside the ear or emerge from your earhole of its own accord

If you suspect your ears are blocked by wax, there are a few telltale signs to look out for, including difficulty hearing, dizziness, itchy ear, tinnitus (a whining sound in the ear) and earache. If you experience any of these it's worth visiting your local pharmacy in the first instance, where you can obtain various drops which help to dissolve blocked wax. If symptoms persist, visit your GP.

SPECIAL TREATMENTS

For many people, earwax build-up will just be a minor annoyance on the odd occasion, but for some it can persist and become more of a problem. In these cases, there are a number of private treatments that can be effective.

✂ Ear irrigation – irrigation of any sort usually involves water, and this is the case with ear irrigation where warm water is injected into the ear canal, often with a large syringe, to flush wax out. Drops are usually administered before this procedure, to make the wax softer and potentially easier to remove. However, in 2017 the National Institute for Health and Care Excellence suggested that irrigation with a syringe can cause permanent damage to the delicate ear drum as the pressure being applied isn't as controlled as it could be. But there is an alternative, which is electronic irrigation. It follows the same principle, using pressurized water, except that it's controlled by a machine.

✂ Microsuction – yes, this involves suction, applied by a medical suction device (a miniature wand-like vacuum) guided by a health professional who is equipped with a microscope to direct the instrument. It is promoted as the safest and most painless way to remove wax from the ears, and the procedure itself takes just a few minutes.

TOP TIP – EARPLUGS

As we mentioned, one of the causes of earwax build-up can be earplugs. Whether you use them for your job or to help you sleep at night, pushing a foreign (albeit soft) object into your ear over a long period can compact wax. The trick is to experiment to find a pair that feel comfortable, insert them gently, and keep them clean (if reusable).

- Well-Being -

Here we get to a subject that you might not expect to find in a book about grooming. 'Well-being' may sound a bit vague, but it's defined (in the *Oxford English Dictionary*) as 'a state of being comfortable, healthy, or happy'. What has this got to do with grooming? Well, we said at the outset that the work you put in to looking good will also have the bonus of making you feel good. Taking care of yourself by crafting your appearance and paying attention to yourself on the outside has a side effect of boosting your self-confidence and sense of worth, and giving you a positive mental attitude. You get a sense that you're doing the best for yourself, even in small, superficial ways. Diet, physical activity and relaxation all add up to good grooming for your mind and your body. This section will look at some of the ways you can do this.

Grooming for Good Health

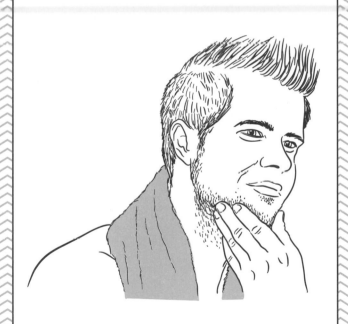

To go back to the car analogy at the beginning of the book, regular maintenance is the key to ensuring everything is working as it should. If you regularly wash your beloved car, you're more likely to notice a new scratch on the paintwork or chip in the windscreen. So, by doing something as basic and superficial as cleaning, you can get a sense of any potential problems, minor and major. On a more positive note, you will also get a buzz out of seeing your car gleaming (especially if you put the extra effort in and wax it). In the same way, giving yourself regular, basic attention by upping your grooming game will help you spot anything that might concern you – that ingrowing toenail, those new grey hairs – and you'll feel better for getting it sorted. And when you're looking your best, you feel better.

There's plenty of evidence to support this idea. The mental health charity Mind suggests that personal care is a key factor in maintaining a positive attitude for life and self-worth. Basically, if you have a lifestyle that involves constructive 'me time' or, 'self-care', you'll be happier.

WHAT IS SELF-CARE?

Practicing self-care is about prioritizing your physical well-being and mental health – essentially, looking after yourself. We often think that, as responsible adults, we naturally have this covered, but the pressure to achieve in our increasingly busy day-to-day lives can mean we put ourselves last. Self-care combines daily acts of maintenance with regular beneficial treats to ensure your body and mind doesn't get too run down.

Grooming is self-care on a small, daily, manageable scale. We're not saying you should book yourself into a week-long spa break (although relaxation is an important part of the whole, as we'll see later on p.171); the point is to recognize that putting time into your appearance, in all the ways we've discussed throughout the book, is a worthwhile endeavor for your overall health and well-being.

TAKING YOUR SELF-CARE GROOMING TO THE NEXT LEVEL

If you really want to ramp up the self-care factor of your grooming routine, and we heartily recommend that you do, here are some ideas:

✂ Take a bath (instead of a shower) once in a while – on a day-to-day basis, a shower is often the most efficient way of washing, but nothing beats a bath for the relaxation factor. Try chilling out with some tunes and taking your time – just remember to wash while you're at it!

✂ Get a haircut at a swanky (or swankier) hairdresser – you might have found a hairdresser that you swear by already; even so, why not push the boat out and try a more exclusive place, or try an added extra from your regular hairdresser, like a professional shave?

✄ Get a manicure/pedicure/facial – knock up your own moisturizer (see p.78) at home or take a trip out and get a treatment to make you feel on top form.

✄ Go for some grooming-related retail therapy – check out a nifty new safety razor or hand-crafted comb, or splash out on some quality shampoos or styling products to expand your grooming arsenal. Another sure-fire way to enhance your mood is to get some new threads. We haven't covered clothes in this book, but making yourself look smart with what you wear is a kind of grooming in itself.

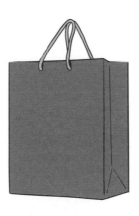

- Food and Drink -

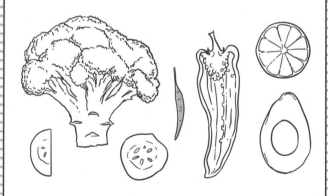

What happens on the inside of your body can directly affect what happens on the outside – and one of the biggest influences you have on what happens on the inside lies in what food and drink you consume. So, when you eat healthily you're doing your body a favour and when you eat badly you're bringing it down. Pretty obvious, right? But did you know that food and drink can affect specific areas of the body? Your hair, nails, skin and teeth can be boosted by certain vitamins and minerals, so if you eat the right things you can actually make your grooming life easier.

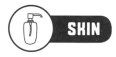 **SKIN**

As we've mentioned already, your skin is basically an organ, and as such it's pretty sensitive. For example, there is research to suggest that what you eat can affect your hormone balance, which in turn can affect your complexion. So even if you're doing everything right by moisturizing, exfoliating, cleansing and protecting your skin, you could still be seeing blemishes. Here's some advice on what you should and shouldn't eat to benefit your skin.

WHAT TO EAT AND DRINK

✂ Water – duh! But seriously, water hydrates your skin, making it look less wrinkled. It might not be the most exciting beverage in the world, but if you learn to love it you'll be doing yourself a world of favors.

✂ Green tea – you might be partial to a brew, but if you drink green tea daily instead of black you'll be making your skin smoother and more elastic, and boosting your skin's resistance to UV light. It's down to polyphenols in the tea, which are antioxidants that combat cell damage and reduce inflammation.

✂ Olive oil – if you don't already cook with olive oil, here's why you should. It contains a high percentage of monounsaturated fatty acids, which sound bad but may actually work to make skin look younger. If you're getting more than two teaspoons a day, you're on the right track – just don't swig it straight from the bottle!

✗ Carrots – some people say they help you see in the dark, but that's what electric lights are for. Instead, eat them because the carotene they contain will give you added yellow tones in your complexion, which will make it look healthier in general.

WHAT TO AVOID

✗ White bread and white rice – they might taste great, but they also contain refined, sugary carbs that increase insulin production in your body and so increase the production of hormones known as androgens. Higher levels of these androgens trigger your skin to release more oil, which means an increased chance of blocked pores.

✗ Cow's milk – milk is believed to be an inflammatory, which means it can aggravate things like rashes and wrinkles.

✂ Fatty foods – sounds like a no-brainer, but fatty foods are bad for your skin as well as your waistline. Higher-fat diets are associated with ageing skin. A study in the *American Journal of Clinical Nutrition* noted that an increase in fat in your diet can up your odds of developing wrinkles.

✂ Alcohol that isn't red wine – yes, it's true. While red wine contains skin-saving antioxidants, there's no such luck for beer, spirits and other types of wine. Alcohol in general will dehydrate the body (and therefore the skin), so all you'll be getting is a tasty tipple and a slight buzz.

HAIR AND NAILS

Your hair and nails might seem like they do their own thing, since they're just made up of unfeeling protein (keratin), but of course they're nourished by your body. So, if you're looking after your body and filling it with goodness, it will be evident in your hair and nails.

WHAT TO EAT AND DRINK

✂ Green vegetables – iron, found in abundance in this sort of veg, is key to boosting the health of hair and nails. Your hair follicles rely on having a rich supply of nutrients delivered to them in the blood, and a lack of iron disrupts the supply. Ensuring you eat lots of vegetables like kale, spinach, broccoli and green salad items means you'll keep your iron topped up and your hair looking nourished.

✂ Oily fish – this is a great source of omega-3 fatty acids, which help to keep your scalp from drying out by creating natural oils in the cells. Omega-3s can't be produced by the body, so taking them in by way of foods such as salmon, mackerel and sardines gives you a big boost. If you don't like fish, you should eat more almonds and walnuts.

✂ Smoothies with Vitamins C, A and E – vitamin C (found in oranges, kiwis, grapefruit and red and green peppers) helps with the absorption of iron (see above); vitamin A (carrots) promotes cell growth and helps with the production of the scalp's natural oil; and vitamin E helps hair growth through aiding blood circulation. It's readily found in avocadoes, which can be easily added to fruit smoothies – check out the recipe below.

✂ Eggs and wholegrains – biotin is a B vitamin (B7) that helps with cell fortification and protein production which strengthens hair and helps it to grow, so it's pretty essential when it comes to healthy hair. You can also get biotin from wholegrain foods like brown rice, oatmeal and wholewheat bread and pasta.

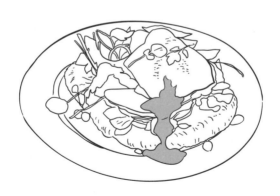

HAIR-BOOSTING SMOOTHIE

Try this follicle-fortifying smoothie for a tasty and quick way to get a few of your five a day and nourish your hair.

Combine the following in a blender and enjoy:

½ avocado – for vitamin E

1 cup spinach – for iron

1 cup strawberries – for vitamin C and E

1 kiwi fruit (peeled) – for vitamin C

1½ cups almond milk – for omega-3s

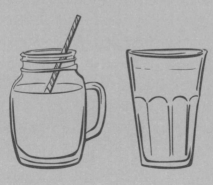

WHAT TO AVOID

 Sweets – by which we mean refined sugar found in all of those little treats you might fancy, the most grown-up of which is probably chocolate. We won't judge you if you still have a soft spot for gummy bears, but you won't be doing your hair any favors by eating them, since the extra insulin that comes with consuming them also increases levels of androgens, which can shrink hair follicles.

 High GI (glycemic index) foods – things like white bread (pizza!), white pasta (spaghetti!), potatoes (chips!) and cake (cake!) are all guaranteed, like the sweets above, to crank up your androgen levels just like refined sugar. So do your best to avoid them.

TOP TIP – MOOD FOOD

You might have heard of the phrase 'hangry' – well, it's a real thing! If, from lack of food, your blood

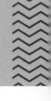

sugar drops below a certain level, you might well feel tired or irritable as a result. The idea is to keep your blood sugar levels steady, so there are no peaks and slumps. To do this you could try to eat smaller (but more regular) portions throughout the day. So, as well as eating the right things for your hair, skin, teeth and nails, spare a thought for your mood – you don't want to add any wrinkles or greys by making yourself hangry.

 TEETH AND MOUTH

What with your gnashers being placed at the beginning of your digestive tract, you can safely presume that they are going to take a bashing from whatever you're eating and drinking throughout the day. They're built to last, of course, so for the most part your food and drink intake won't have a negative impact on your teeth, but there are certain things that will. The same goes for the mouth itself.

WHAT TO EAT AND DRINK

✂ Cheese – nothing to do with saying 'cheese' when posing for a photo, but rather this dairy product is a big boost to the health of teeth since it contains calcium, which strengthens enamel. However, it's also quite acidic, which means that it could lower the pH in your mouth, which is not beneficial. Although the extra chewing involved will produce more saliva to neutralize this acid, take care and eat cheese in moderation.

✂ Apples – this fruit is sweet but it's also alkaline, meaning it won't encourage any excess acid in your mouth. What it will do, though, is produce lots of saliva in your mouth, which will help carry away bacteria. The fact that apples often take some chewing to break down means they will stimulate your gums as you munch.

✂ Non-dairy milk – it's true that cow's milk packs the biggest punch when it comes to teeth-strengthening calcium, but, as we said earlier, it's not great for your skin. So you should consider non-dairy milks, since they are often fortified with almost as much calcium as your moo juice. Soy milk contains isoflavones, proven to reduce the risk of heart disease, and almond milk is rich in vitamin E, which makes for healthy skin.

✂ Veg juice – this might not sound like the most exciting thing in the world to drink, but juices containing green vegetables will help to fight against gum disease. The key thing to watch out for (if you're buying them) is too much fruit or any added sugar, since that will end up doing more harm than good.

TOP TIP – BLENDER OR JUICER?

If all you want to do is make smoothies and soups and whizz stuff up for cooking, a blender has got you covered. But making juice isn't as easy as just blitzing a load of oranges – you need to extract the pulp so the end product is smooth and drinkable (unless you enjoy chewing your juice). So if you're thinking about investing in a machine to boost your fruit and veg intake, go for a combo blender/juicer, which will be useful in everyday cooking as well as for delicious juices.

WHAT TO AVOID

✂ Sugary and acidic drinks – you've known from an early age that sugary drinks are bad for your teeth, so they should really only be an occasional treat. However, it's worth noting that fruit juices can be just as bad – especially ones with lots of citric acid (orange, grapefruit, etc.) – so these too should either be a treat or drunk with a meal, i.e. not on their own, so the effect is diffused.

✂ Chewy and sticky foods – apart from being really annoying to eat, the kind of foods that are likely to get lodged in your teeth (like dried fruit, for instance) are a danger since, by hanging around in the mouth longer, they will result in increased acid production, which is not good for your mouth. To combat this you could chew some sugar-free gum, which will promote saliva and thus neutralize the acid.

✂ Coffee and alcohol – you might consider one or both of these to be essential to getting through a day/week, but you will also be aware that neither, in excess, is healthy. Both drinks dry your mouth out, reducing the amount of saliva, which is necessary to cleanse the mouth of leftover food.

- Exercise -

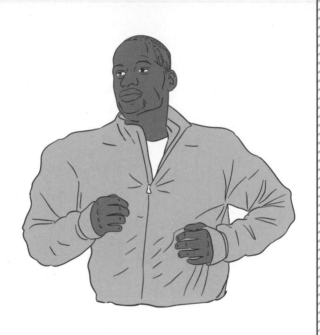

What has exercise got to do with the state of your hair and skin, you say? Plenty! You might be thinking, exercise equals sweat, which is surely a negative when it comes to skin health, but you'd be wrong. Exercise also increases blood flow around the body, meaning molecules important for hair and skin health are delivered more readily. There are some pitfalls, though – being outside in bad weather, for example, is going to be harrowing for your skin, and all swimmers know what chlorine does to their hair. This chapter will take you through some of the best ways to factor in exercise while being conscious of your grooming habits.

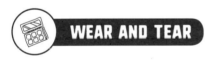 **WEAR AND TEAR**

Regular exercise is one of the best things you can do for your body, but it comes with its own risks attached, depending on the type of activity you choose. We'll start by taking a look at some of the potential problem areas, to help you decide which kind of exercise you might want to avoid.

POTENTIAL PROBLEM AREAS

Hair:

- Increased washing after exercise will wash away natural oils
- Exposure to the elements (sun, wind, rain, cold) can cause damage
- Exposure to synthetic chemicals (e.g. chlorine) can cause damage

Face:

- Exposure to the elements (sun, wind, rain, cold) can cause damage
- Trapped water in the ears can trigger an infection
- Lips are especially prone to cracking when exposed to low temperatures

Body:

- More exertion means more sweat and more body odor (if you don't wash properly)
- Nipples can be damaged when friction is involved in your exercise (e.g. running)

Hands:

- Blisters, callouses and other skin damage can result during exercise that involves the use of the hands (e.g. racquet sports)

Groin:

- Chafing can be an issue when friction is involved (e.g. cycling)

Feet:

- Public facilities (e.g. showers and changing rooms) can be the source of bacterial infections
- Blisters, callouses and other skin damage can result during exercise that involves high-intensity use of the feet (e.g. hiking, running)
- Increased levels of sweat can invite skin irritation and issues like athlete's foot

So what can you do to avoid giving your skin and hair a hard time while you exercise? Below we've organized activities into three categories: low-, mid- and high-impact exercise. The impact being the amount of stress you'll potentially be putting your 'groom zones' under.

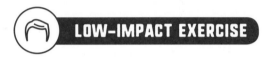

LOW-IMPACT EXERCISE

These could be indoor activities that are also low-impact on your body in general, which means you'll still get an exercise fix, but you'll be taking it easy on yourself. The slight downside is that with some of these activities you might not get as much of an aerobic buzz, but that might strike the right balance for you.

Yoga – this indoor activity is all about control – of your breath and of the body and the energy inside it – so it can provide a slow but significant anaerobic workout which will help tone your body (and so your skin). The poses it involves will increase suppleness from head to toe, and some types of yoga (Balayam, for example) are akin to acupuncture, where pressure is applied, which increases blood flow and so benefits hair and nails especially. You'll also find yoga to be great for de-stressing, which means you'll be feeling great too.

TOP TIP – YOGA FOR HAIR GROWTH

One of the simplest yoga poses which will help with digestion/nutrient dispersal and blood flow to the upper part of your body is the 'diamond' or 'Vajrasana' pose. It's as simple as sitting on your feet, heels and feet cupping your butt, with a straight back. Your hands can rest on your thighs, near your knees, with palms up. There are many more poses which increase blood flow specifically to the head, but these tend to be more advanced, so if you like the idea of them, why not join a local yoga class?

Gym – today, gyms are full of different equipment and as such can be costly, but even the most budget-friendly gym will have something for you to walk or jog lightly on, or perform a few steady leg and arm exercises on. The main benefit, in terms of grooming, is that you're indoors, so the elements aren't taking it out on you. If you stick to exercises like walking on the treadmill, using the step climber and light strength training with weights, you'll be able to work up a sweat without too much stress.

T'ai chi – this exercise is so chilled out it looks like you're in slow motion (and you are!). Another ancient practice that is about careful control of body and energy, it is believed t'ai chi helps with aerobic capacity and muscle strength. So if you do want to ramp up your regime, combining it with something relaxed like this is a winner. It even helps reduce inflammation and boosts your immune system. On a fine day in China, you'll see people doing t'ai chi in the park, but classes are more often indoors, away from the disquieting elements.

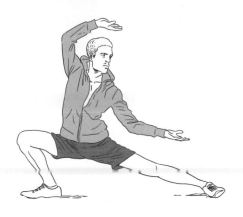

 MID-IMPACT EXERCISE

Cycling – the great thing about cycling is that you can make it as high- or low-impact as you like. You could do a few steady miles along a nice cycle path each weekend when the weather is fair or commit to full Lycra and crank out the miles in all weather. There are accessories for every part of your body for all possible weather conditions, so if you're concerned about damaging your hair or skin, chances are you can fend off the elements one way or another. Wear sunblock in the summer, moisturize before your ride in the winter and apply anti-chafe chamois cream before epic rides. If you cycle regularly, there will be times when you can't beat the weather and you'll feel the impact of the sun, rain or cold, but if you consider the health benefits you might agree that it's worth it. (You could always use an exercise bike, but you'll miss out on the fresh air and outside stimulation.) Cycling, as with any moderate exercise, increases blood flow and so will ramp up the nourishment available to hair and nails. It also helps your immune system by increasing the circulation of antibodies, which means any ailments that might affect the condition of your skin will be warded off more regularly.

Running – as with cycling, there are lots of accessories available to allow you to participate in all weather conditions, so you can gain some protection, despite it being a largely outdoor activity. (Yes, you could go to the gym and pound the treadmill, but the exhilaration factor will be lost and the boredom factor high.) Once again, you can ramp the intensity up or down, depending on if you choose to shuffle or sprint, and the advantage of running over cycling is that you don't have to shell out for a bike. There are various precautions to take, though, since it is just your body vs the tarmac. Friction on the nipples (why do men still have them?) can be an issue on prolonged runs, and of course there is a concentrated amount of stress in the knees (which won't affect your look but might make you walk a bit funny!). How much you sweat will depend on your DNA, but if you do find that you perspire a lot, which can have pore-blocking effects, you can apply dry shampoo to your hair and scalp, and baking soda, which is antibacterial, for an additional moisture-absorbing effect on any other part of your body.

GO *NATUREL* – WALKING

A gentle stroll is a pleasant, low-key way to get some exercise, but you can also strap on your proper walking gear and cover some serious miles. Either way, you'll be stepping the speed and intensity down a notch and hopefully experiencing nature and pleasing scenery. As opposed to running or cycling, this is much more of a relaxing way to get physical. You'll also be taking in vitamin D from exposure to sunlight, which is known to boost the health of bones and teeth and support your immune system – but don't forget the sunscreen if it's hot!

Ball games – chasing a ball around a court, field or pitch is something most of us have done at one time or another, even if the last time was PE in high school. But sports like football, baseball, tennis and basketball are long-loved classics and as such there are likely to be facilities and clubs near you. (You'll notice we didn't include heavy contact sports, which, as wonderful as they are, are not known for being kind to your skin/face/hair/anything.) Many of them involve running, which will give you an aerobic workout, and most, if not all, of them can be played indoors when the weather is truly awful.

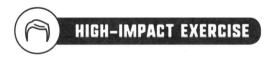

HIGH-IMPACT EXERCISE

Being adventurous and testing yourself might be your kind of thing, in which case you might well be into sports like surfing, snowboarding or rock climbing. These are the kinds of physical activities which often require specialist equipment and extensive travel, so they're by no means as common as some of the sports mentioned above. But they do come with an incredible amount of excitement and an incomparable buzz. But, of course, they also come with incomparable detrimental effects for hair and skin. Seawater might give your hair a unique look, but it will also leave it dry and brittle, as the salt draws out moisture. Combined with exposure to the sun, this is bad news. We've already covered how winter temperatures damage your skin, so naturally this applies when you're out on the slopes. And as for scaling rock faces, cramming hands and feet into tight, sharp-edged crevices – need we say more?

Swimming – it's hailed as one of the best all-round exercises you can do, but public pools are not always a haven for good health. Aside from the sometimes less-than-sanitary changing areas, chlorinated water is irritating to your eyes and will dry out your hair and skin. And the extra showering involved will also be washing away oils. However, there are such things as goggles and caps, so be sure to wear them if you want to partake.

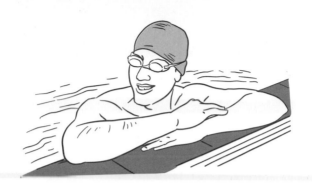

GETTING PROPERLY KITTED OUT

It might sound vain, but your workout outfit is pretty important. Not just because you want to look cool at the gym or out in the park (although that can never hurt), but because improper clothing can cause a number of problems. If you just slap on any old sweatshirt and shorts you'll quickly find that they will be impeding your progress in one way or another – too baggy, too bulky, too warm, etc. If you're exercising in clothes like this you're inviting sweat to build up unnecessarily and encouraging chafing of all kinds to occur. Take the time to choose and invest in sport-specific clothes that will treat your body right (for example, cycling and running clothing is often made of material which has a wicking effect, drawing sweat away from the skin). You'll be much happier as a result.

TO BATHE OR NOT TO BATHE?

We've talked a lot about how bathing can sometimes have negative effects for your hair and skin, so you might be tempted to ask, do I really need to shower after my workout? While it's true that excessive bathing will not do your skin and hair any favors, sweat that remains on the skin will promote bacteria proliferation, which itself can lead to rashes and other blemishes. So, keep it quick, keep it tepid, but keep it in your routine!

Rest and - Relaxation -

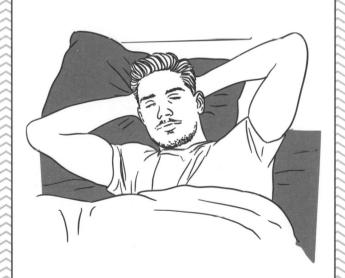

Ever heard the phrase 'beauty sleep'? Well, as unbelievable as this notion sounds, apparently it's real! The proper amount of sleep genuinely makes you look better, just like the improper amount makes you look awful. This chapter looks at the various ways rest and relaxation can help you in your grooming efforts – and who doesn't want to make time for more of that in their life?

TOP TIP - HOW MUCH SLEEP?

A common question is, 'How much sleep should I be getting?' People often quote 8 hours as the standard, but it's not a one-size fits all deal. To get an idea of how much sleep you need, simply note how you're feeling once you've woken up and started your day. If you wake up feeling tired and spend the day thinking 'I could do with a nap', you should try going to bed earlier. It's also about the quality of sleep (i.e. sound, uninterrupted sleep), so consider earplugs (but see p.178), an eye mask or blackout curtains if you're constantly waking up.

SLEEP AND YOUR SKIN

Sleep gives your body an opportunity to revive itself in all sorts of ways. Your brain is still active and is busy consolidating memories and new skills you've learned, your immune system is being boosted by the production of extra proteins and your blood pressure is reduced. But there's also plenty of activity in your skin.

✂ Drying out – for all the good that sleep does, it also has the less-than-helpful effect of drying out your skin a little during the night. The reasons behind this are that your skin becomes more acidic, and at the same time is less saturated by the natural oils your skin produces throughout the day (but less so at night). This means you lose more moisture while you're asleep, and so your skin dries out. However, you can counteract this by applying a night-time moisturizer, which often contains more potent moisturizing ingredients like retinols.

✂ Cell regeneration – on the plus side, night-time is the natural period for skin cells to be dividing and so repairing. This is also a great time to be applying skin-replenishing products, because your cells will be more receptive to it.

✂ Cortisol reduction – daily activities often involve stress of one sort or another, which produces a hormone called cortisol. This encourages inflammation in the skin, but when you're asleep you're protected because you're not producing that extra cortisol.

✂ Slim down – there might not be any special processes happening that are magically making you thinner overnight, but it's been proven that people who get a healthy amount of sleep are less likely to be obese. It is believed that sleep-deprived people have less of a chemical called leptin, which is responsible for making us feel full, while simultaneously having higher levels of ghrelin, which stimulates appetite.

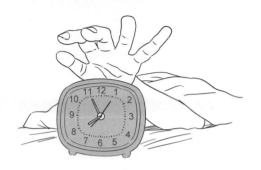

LACK OF SLEEP
(AND THE DAMAGE IT CAN DO)

Now let's take a look at what a lack of sleep can do to your body. Aside from adversely affecting your skin, sleep deprivation can have a whole host of negative effects, including difficulty in concentrating (which might just be an annoyance for work, but it could be a danger for driving), a reduction in sex drive (depending on your normal libido this could be more devastating for some than for others), high blood pressure, increased risk of diabetes and heart attack (if you experience full-blown insomnia), as well as irritability and delirium. So, it's safe to say that sleep is one of the most essential factors in a healthy lifestyle.

HOW TO IMPROVE YOUR SLEEP

There are things you can do in the daytime as well as at night to improve the quality of your sleep. Here are a few ideas:

✂ Lose the booze – alcohol might relax you, but it also disturbs your sleep as you experience what are essentially withdrawal symptoms as you slumber.

Avoid drinking at least 4 hours before bed. The same goes for caffeine.

✂ Remove the phones and tablets – you might like to read while you're in bed, and you might well use a tablet or phone to do it, but this is not good for your sleep. The light emitted by most screens is known as blue light, which the brain reads as daylight and so gets geared up for action instead of winding down. You might use your phone as an alarm, but if you want a proper night's rest, consider leaving it on charge downstairs and relying on an alarm clock.

✂ Get the temperature right – it goes without saying that a room that is too hot or too cold will inhibit sleep. The ideal temperature is around 18°C (64°F). You can also make the room more hospitable by opening a window to let some fresh air in an hour before bedtime – just keep an eye on the temperature if you do.

✂ Get the light right – the last thing you want before bed is a bright light relaying the message to your brain that it's not in fact night-time. Most people have bedside lamps, but even these can be too bright if they're large and have a high-watt bulb. Opt for something small or something that has a dimmer to really get the light down to a minimum. Blackout curtains will ensure summer sun and streetlights are prevented from disturbing you.

✂ Reduce the noise – if your partner snores it can be a nightmare, but the same goes for traffic noise, seagulls, clocks that are ticking too loudly – they can all set your mind into action or annoyance mode. Some noises you can get used to (especially if you live in a city where background noise is a constant) but if you struggle to drop off at bedtime, the most obvious answer is earplugs. As we've mentioned, it's essential to keep reusable plugs clean, and even then you might notice wax building up. The key is to find a type that stay put while you sleep, are comfortable and have as little impact on the health of your ear as possible. Ideally, earplugs will be a temporary crutch for you, as opposed to a long-term solution, since weeks of plugging your ears can cause problems of its own.

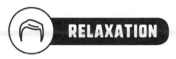 **RELAXATION**

HOW STRESS CAN AFFECT THE BODY

Making relaxation a part of our average day is becoming ever more rare. Everyone's routine is different, but can you honestly say that you would struggle to find 10 minutes here or there to drop what you're doing and relax in one way or another? The first hurdle is a mental one – admitting that, in reality, you *do* have the time for it and you *should* spend time doing it.

You might think that you've got yourself together and you're strong enough to take a bit of punishment from the daily demands of your life, but the fact is that stress of any sort is bad not only for your mind but also for your body – even your looks. Stress is known to contribute to various conditions that lead to hair loss, including *trichotillomania* (literally pulling your hair out, but without always realizing it), *alopecia areata* (the sudden loss of small amounts of hair from the head) and *telogen effluvium* (increased shedding of hair in the natural way). These are all more extreme examples, but if you let stress get a small foothold, there's no telling if it will escalate. Your skin, of course, is also affected. As we've mentioned, stress hormones cause inflammation, which can cause acne. When your body is stressed it's in fight-or-flight mode, which means blood flow is directed to muscles, prepping them for action, instead of to areas like the scalp where it has a nourishing effect. If you use alcohol to take the edge off your stress you're in danger of dehydrating yourself, as well as encouraging redness in the cheeks, which is never attractive.

In short, once you get that stress ball rolling, it's easy for it to gather speed, which might leave you in a bit of a mess. That is, unless you take a little time to level yourself out.

MAKING DE-STRESSING A PART OF EVERY DAY

Grooming is about taking some time out for you, and this must apply to your mind as well as your body. Here are some ideas for little ways to make any day a little less stressful:

✗ Breathe – you can do this exercise wherever you are. Take a few consecutive deep, slow breaths in through your nose and out through your mouth. Concentrate solely on the feeling of the air moving in and out. The oxygen boost will act to reduce stress by putting your body at ease, and the act of relaxed concentration and simple focus will calm your mind.

✗ Walk – regardless of where you work, you should always get out on your lunch break and get moving. Yes, you might be desperately busy, but just 10 minutes of walking can promote stress-busting endorphins to circulate within the body. If nothing else, it will give you a physical and mental break from the task that has you so engrossed.

X Snack – a healthy one, of course! Bananas are a great source of potassium, which helps regulate blood pressure (which is obviously peaking when you're stressed out). You can also try eating 'mindfully' which means focusing on the act of eating and the sensations that are happening – the taste, the smell, the texture – as opposed to scoffing it while you type out an email.

Last Word

In many ways, grooming is a stress-busting, feel-good activity in its own right, so by expanding your routine to include more things that make you look and feel good you're getting an automatic win. It's a positive lifestyle choice that might seem time-consuming and expensive at first, but will ultimately repay you with improvements to your physical and mental health – not to mention general positivity and happiness in your day-to-day life. The best part is you can take your time and expand your routine at your own pace, trying new things here and there to find what works for you and what you do and don't enjoy. Grooming requires a little commitment, but it's nothing you can't take back or change – that beard is only a trim and a safety-razor shave away from disappearing – so try out some new ideas and groom your way to better health and happiness.

GLOSSARY OF TERMS

alopecia areata – also known as 'spot baldness'. A condition whereby a person will develop bald spots (on the head and in other areas).

androgens – male hormones (such as testosterone) that contribute to sexual maturity in young men and balding and sebaceous-gland activity in adult men.

anti-shine powder – a cosmetic powder that can be applied to the face to reduce the visibility of oily skin.

beard balm/oil – a preparation (oil or oil-based balm) applied to facial hair and skin as a moisturizer.

blepharoplasty – medical term to describe surgical alterations to the eyelid and other skin around the eye.

Botox – a procedure whereby *Botulinum* toxin is injected into the muscles (often the face) to reduce the appearance of wrinkles, lines and other signs of skin ageing.

brittle nail syndrome – a condition whereby the nail plate is abnormally brittle and prone to chipping and splitting.

bronzer – a cosmetic product (a powder or a liquid)

applied to the skin to give it a 'bronze' look, imitating a suntan.

brow powder – a cosmetic product (a colored waxy powder) applied to the eyebrows to give them a fuller look.

buzz cut – a very closely-cropped hairstyle created with electric hair clippers.

cartridge razor – a wet-shave razor that uses disposable blade cartridges, that can be replaced easily by slotting them into place onto a razor 'stem'.

clay – a thick, opaque, often creamy hairstyling product that contains an element of clay and adds body to your hair.

cleanser – a skincare product that is specially formulated to remove pollutants from the pores.

concealer – a skin-colored cosmetic product, often a thick liquid, applied to the skin to disguise the appearance of blemishes.

cream – a thick but loose hairstyling product that adds moisture and shine to your hair with a low to medium hold.

cuticle – a dead layer of skin that occurs just beyond the point where your finger skin ends and your nail begins.

dental pick – a narrow, hook-type implement for cleaning between teeth and scraping plaque.

dermal filler – a substance (e.g. collagen injected into the skin (dermis) to 'fill out' the appearance of wrinkles and other signs of ageing.

double-edged razor (also safety razor) – a wet-shaving razor designed to be used with a traditional, single double-edged razor blade, which is inserted into the head of the razor.

ear irrigation – a process by which warm water is injected into the ear canal, often with a large syringe, to flush wax out.

eczema – a skin condition characterized by widespread red, cracked, itchy blotches that can 'flare up' at different times and as a result of different irritants.

emery board – a nail file, usually consisting of a strip of card or wood coated in fine grains of abrasive emery (corundite).

fibre – a thick, slightly sticky styling product that gives medium hold.

finishing product – hairstyling products, such as hairspray, that are used to 'finish' your styling efforts by fixing the hair in place or by adding shine or de-frizzing.

foundation – a skin-colored liquid or powder that can be applied to the skin to create a more even tone and smooth appearance.

fringe – a haircut/style that consists of hair covering, or partially covering, the forehead.

gel – a viscous, sometimes clear or semi-clear styling product that gives high hold.

GI – Glycaemic Index. A rating system, given in figures, for foods containing carbohydrates. The figure shown is proportionate to the speed at which carbohydrates in the food in question are converted to sugars. High GI foods (having a higher GI number) include white bread, potatoes and white rice.

gynecomastia – enlargement of the male breast tissue (glandular tissue, fatty tissue or skin). A common name for the condition is 'man boobs' or 'moobs'.

hair mask – a haircare product, often a cream, that is applied to washed, dry hair in order to add moisture. It is removed after a short period of time by rinsing the hair.

hangnail – a protruding shard of skin (as opposed to a piece of nail) at the end of the finger, near the nail.

hyperpigmentation – a skin condition that manifests as darker areas on the skin, caused by excess melanin production.

hypoallergenic – defines a cosmetic or skincare product as 'suitable for sensitive skin'.

interdental brush – a small brush, consisting mostly of a needle-like head covered in fine bristles, designed to be used to clean between individual teeth.

manscaping – a collective term describing the act of grooming, especially of body hair.

microdermabrasion – an exfoliation procedure involving the use of mildly abrasive crystals to buff the skin and remove dead cells.

microsuction – a method of removing excess ear wax by inserting a wand-like vacuum into the ears.

minoxidil (e.g. Rogaine) – a topical medicine used to treat hair loss.

mousse – a light, foamy hairstyling product that provides a high hold once set.

omega-3 fatty acids – polyunsaturated fatty acids which cannot be synthesized by the body; therefore, their intake through digestion of certain foods is beneficial to the body.

paste – a dense but smooth hairstyling product that gives medium hold and a matte finish.

pomade – an oil- or water-based hairstyling product that gives a low to medium hold and a high shine, especially suited for combed-in styles.

psoriasis – a skin condition characterized by widespread red, cracked, itchy patches covered by scaly skin.

putty – a smooth, thick hairstyling product that gives medium hold and a matte finish.

quiff/pompadour – a haircut/style defined by a peaked wave of hair at the front of the head, and either brushed-flat or shaved-back hair at the sides, as made famous by celebrities like Elvis Presley and Johnny Cash.

razor bumps – ingrown hairs that have occurred as a result of shaving, causing tiny abscesses.

razor burn – redness in the skin and hair follicles as a result of being irritated by the blade of a shaving razor.

relaxer – a hairstyling product formulated to 'relax' tightly curled hair so it can be managed more easily and styled in a straighter fashion.

rhinoplasty – cosmetic surgery undertaken to reshape the nose.

Rogaine – see minoxidil.

rosacea – a skin condition characterized by long-lasting redness in the face, which may also involve increased visibility of blood vessels and a stinging sensation.

safety razor – see double-edged razor.

sebaceous glands – small glands responsible for secreting sebum (see below) into the hair and skin.

sebum – natural oil secreted by the sebaceous glands to nourish hair and skin.

self-care – the practice of combining daily acts of maintenance with regular beneficial treats to ensure one's body and mind don't get too run down.

stratum corneum – the outermost layer of the skin.

telogen effluvium – a scalp disorder characterized by increased shedding of hair from the head.

toner – most often a water-based skincare product formulated to hydrate and clarify the skin.

tongue scraper – a small plastic implement used to clean the tongue by scraping along its surface.

trichotillomania – a nervous disorder whereby the sufferer unconsciously pulls out strands of their own hair.

unibrow – a common name for when eyebrows have not been groomed to the extent they meet in the middle, above the nose, forming a single ('uni') brow.

veneer – custom-made ceramic coverings that resemble natural teeth, used to create a literal veneer over the front of an unsightly tooth.

wax – a wax-based hairstyling product that offers a high to medium hold.

xerosis – the medical name for dry skin.

If you're interested in finding out more
about our books, find us on Facebook at
Summersdale Publishers and follow us
on Twitter at @Summersdale.

www.summersdale.com

IMAGE CREDITS